OBGYN Meds Made Easy

Callie Parker

Copyright

Copyright © 2025 by Callie Parker

All rights reserved.

No portion of this book may be reproduced in any form without written permission from the publisher or author, except as permitted by U.S. copyright law.

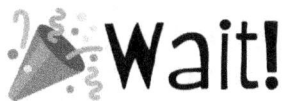 # Wait!

Before You Dive In... Grab Your FREE Nursing Study Survival Kit!

Nursing school is no joke—that's why MadeEasy.Academy is committed to sending the ladder back down and rescuing those of you in the trenches!

Ready to study smarter, not harder? We've got exactly what you need.

Your FREE NCLEX in My Sleep Bundle Includes:

✅ Who's Dying First? The Prioritization Playbook: Because patient safety is kind of a big deal. 😏
✅ Flashcard Frenzy: Memorize or Die Trying: Pre-made Anki cards to save your sanity.
✅ WTF Does This Lab Value Mean? Cheat Sheet: No more second-guessing normal vs. "oh sh*t" levels.
✅ NCLEX Mnemonics That Stick (Like Tape on an IV Line): Memory hacks you'll actually remember.
✅ Med Math Without the Mental Breakdown: Because no one wants to commit a dosage error. 😬

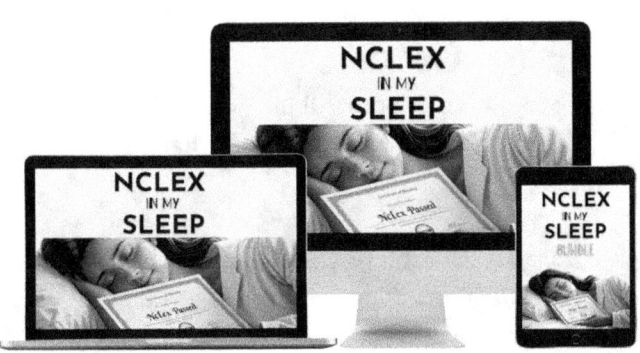

Head over to MadeEasy.Academy to grab your bundle. Let's turn nursing school stress into success!

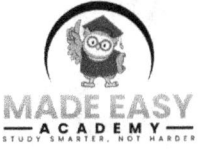

But that's not all...

🎁 BONUS 🎁

Your Bundle Includes an Exclusive 50% OFF Discount Code for your next course at Made Easy Academy
(Launching June 1!)

At MadeEasy.Academy, we don't just simplify nursing—we transform it into an effortless, memorable study process.

For each topic, you'll follow our step by step success guide:

 Step 1. Grab your cheat sheet: All key points, zero fluff.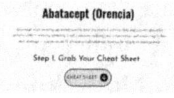

Step 2. Read your mnemonic poem: Clever rhymes to make information stick.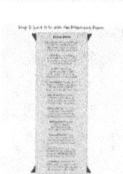

Step 3. Take your fill-in-the-blank quiz: Test your recall without the overwhelm.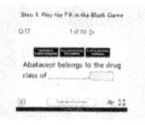

Step 4. Complete your NCLEX challenge: Realistic practice questions with clear rationales.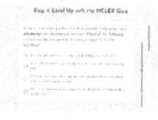

 Step 5. Walk Into the NCLEX Like a Boss: Confident, prepared, and ready to pass.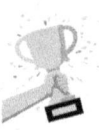

Right now, we're laser-focused on Pharmacology, but we'll soon expand into other crucial nursing topics! Have a topic you want us to cover next? Shoot us an email at hello@madeeasy.academy—we've got you!

TABLE OF CONTENTS

Made Easy: Why and How
Pharmacology Mind Maps
Pharmacology Mind Map Template
Pharmacology Mnemonics

Acetaminophen (Tylenol) 1
Acyclovir (Zovirax) 2
Albuterol (ProAir, Ventolin, Proventil) 3
Amoxicillin (Amoxil) 4
Amoxicillin/Clavulanate (Augmentin) 5
Ampicillin (Principen) 6
Anastrozole (Arimidex) 7
Aspirin (Low-Dose, 81 mg) 8
Atenolol (Tenormin) 9
Azithromycin (Zithromax) 10
Benzocaine (Americaine, Dermoplast) 11
Bupropion (Wellbutrin, Zyban) 12
Calcium Carbonate (Tums, Caltrate) 13
Carbetocin (Duratocin) 14
Carboprost Tromethamine (Hemabate) 15
Cefotaxime (Claforan) 16
Cefotetan (Cefotan) 17
Ceftriaxone (Rocephin) 18
Cephalexin (Keflex) 19
Cetirizine (Zyrtec) 20
Citalopram (Celexa) 21
Clindamycin (Cleocin) 22
Clomiphene Citrate (Clomid, Serophene) 23
Clotrimazole (Lotrimin, Mycelex, Gyne-Lotrimin) 24
Codeine/Acetaminophen (Tylenol #3, #4) 25
Combined Oral Contraceptives (COCs) 26
Conjugated Estrogens (Premarin) 27
Copper IUD (Paragard) 28
Desogestrel 29
Dexamethasone (Decadron) 30
Diclofenac (Voltaren, Cataflam) 31
Dinoprostone (Cervidil, Prepidil, Prostin E2) 32
Diphenhydramine (Benadryl) 33
Docusate Sodium (Colace) 34
Doxycycline 35
Doxylamine/Pyridoxine (Diclegis, Bonjesta) 36
Drospirenone and Ethinyl Estradiol   (Yaz, Yasmin) 37
Duloxetine (Cymbalta) 38
Enoxaparin (Lovenox) 39
Erythromycin (Ery-Tab, E.E.S., Erythrocin) 40

Escitalopram (Lexapro)	41
Estradiol	42
Estradiol Cypionate / Medroxyprogesterone Acetate (Lunelle)	43
Estradiol Transdermal Patch (Climara, Vivelle-Dot, Minivelle)	44
Estradiol Vaginal Insert (Vagifem, Imvexxy)	45
Estradiol Vaginal Ring (Estring, Femring)	46
Estradiol Valerate (Delestrogen)	47
Ethinyl Estradiol/Levonorgestrel	48
Ethinyl Estradiol/Norethindrone	49
Ethinyl Estradiol/Norgestimate (Ortho Tri-Cyclen, Sprintec)	50
Etonogestrel Implant (Nexplanon)	51
Famciclovir (Famvir)	52
Fluconazole (Diflucan)	53
Fluconazole Vaginal Tablet	54
Fluoxetine (Prozac)	55
Folic Acid (Vitamin B9)	56
Gabapentin (Neurontin)	57
Gonadotropins (e.g., FSH, LH, hCG)	58
Hydralazine (Apresoline)	59
Heparin	60
Hydrocodone/Acetaminophen (Norco, Vicodin, Lortab)	61
Hydroxyzine (Vistaril, Atarax)	62
Ibuprofen	63
Indomethacin (Indocin)	64
Insulin	65
Iron Supplements (Ferrous Sulfate, Ferrous Gluconate, etc.)	66
Labetalol (Trandate)	67
Lamotrigine (Lamictal)	68
Letrozole (Femara)	69
Leuprolide (Lupron)	70
Levonorgestrel	71
Levothyroxine (Synthroid, Levoxyl, Euthyrox)	72
Lidocaine (Xylocaine)	73
Loratadine (Claritin)	74
Magnesium Sulfate	75
Medroxyprogesterone Acetate (Depo-Provera)	76
Medroxyprogesterone (Oral – Provera)	77
Mefenamic Acid (Ponstel)	78
Metformin (Glucophage)	79
Methyldopa (Aldomet)	80
Methylergonovine (Methergine)	81
Metoclopramide (Reglan)	82
Metronidazole (Flagyl)	83
Miconazole (Monistat)	84
Misoprostol (Cytotec)	85
Naproxen (Aleve, Naprosyn)	86
Nifedipine (Procardia)	87

Nitrofurantoin (Macrobid, Macrodantin) 88
Norethindrone 89
Norethisterone Enantate (Net-En) 90
Ondansetron (Zofran) 91
Ormeloxifene (Centchroman / Saheli) 92
Oxycodone/Acetaminophen (Percocet) 93
Oxytocin (Pitocin) 94
Paroxetine (Paxil) 95
Penicillin V (Pen-Vee K) 96
Pramoxine 97
Progesterone (Prometrium) 98
Promethazine (Phenergan) 99
Psyllium (Metamucil) 100
Raloxifene (Evista) 101
Rho(D) Immune Globulin (RhoGAM) 102
Sertraline (Zoloft) 103
Simethicone (Gas-X, Mylicon) 104
Sulfamethoxazole/Trimethoprim   (Bactrim, Septra) 105
Tamoxifen (Nolvadex) 106
Terbutaline (Brethine) 107
Terconazole (Terazol) 108
Testosterone (AndroGel, Depo-Testosterone) 109
Topiramate (Topamax) 110
Tranexamic Acid (Lysteda, Cyklokapron) 111
Ulipristal Acetate (Ella) 112
Valacyclovir (Valtrex) 113
Venlafaxine (Effexor, Effexor XR) 114
Vitamin D (Cholecalciferol / Ergocalciferol) 115

WHY Made Easy Works

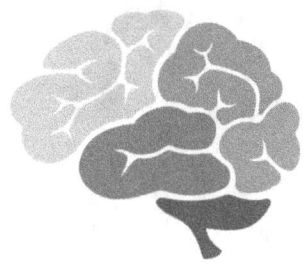

Backed by Brain Science

Let's face it — nursing school can feel like trying to drink from a firehose. Between the jargon, the never-ending lists, and the sheer volume of information, it's easy to feel overwhelmed. That's exactly why the Made Easy series was born: to make the hard stuff stick without frying your brain. And while it might look fun and playful on the outside (hello, rhymes!), it's all built on rock-solid research from the nerdy world of educational psychology.

1. COGNITIVE LOAD THEORY

First up: Cognitive Load Theory. Fancy name, simple idea — your brain can only handle so much at once. When materials are too dense or packed with fluff, your working memory taps out. Educational psychologist John Sweller figured this out, and we took notes. That's why our poems give you the essentials only, in small, memorable doses. Less clutter, more clarity. (Sweller, 1988; Clark et al., 2006)

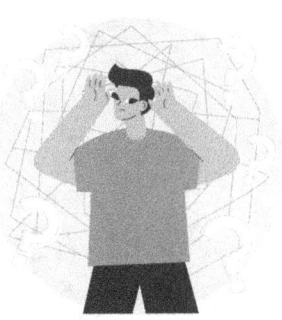

2. DUAL CODING THEORY

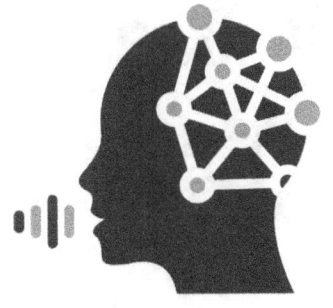

Then there's Dual Coding Theory, brought to us by Allan Paivio. He discovered that we remember things better when we learn them through both words and visuals. Our poems lean into this by using rhyme and rhythm to boost verbal memory — and bolded key terms, color coding, and clean formatting to give your visual brain a treat. Two paths to your brain = double the retention. (Paivio, 1986; Mayer, 2009)

3. ADVANCE ORGANIZERS

Psychologist David Ausubel believed that when we know how new info fits into what we already know, we learn faster. That's the beauty of our repeatable poem structure. Once you get the hang of the format, your brain relaxes — and focuses on what actually matters: the content. Think of it like a familiar playlist for your mind. (Ausubel, 1960)

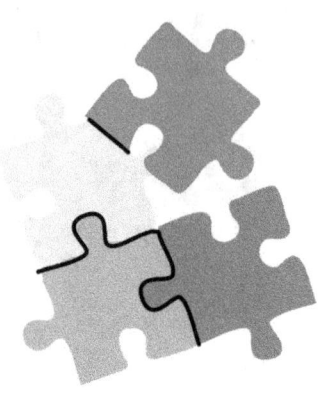

4. MICROLEARNING

Our poems are also bite-sized by design, and that's no accident. Welcome to the world of microlearning — the idea that small, focused learning units are easier to digest and retain. This is a game-changer for busy, burnt-out students. Instead of cramming for hours, you can study just one medication, one skill, or one critical concept at a time. Snack-sized studying with full-course impact. (Hug, 2005; van den Berg & van den Berg, 2021)

5. SPACED REPETITION & RETRIEVAL PRACTICE

Last but definitely not least: spaced repetition and retrieval practice. These two learning powerhouses have proven time and again that the more often you recall information over time, the longer you'll remember it. Our poems are made for this. Easy to reread, perfect for flashcards, and fun enough to come back to (yes, we admitted it). Rinse and repeat — and retain. (Dunlosky et al., 2013)

So, yes — this method might look different than your typical textbook grind. That's the point. It's effective on purpose. Because learning tough topics shouldn't feel impossible. It should feel doable. Even a little fun. And with Made Easy, it totally is.

Read it. Rhyme it. Remember it.

That's the Made Easy Method—a simple but powerful approach to mastering complex nursing material.

ONE — START WITH THE BIG PICTURE

Before diving into individual medications, review the Mind Maps (via QR code). These quick-reference visuals give you the foundational understanding needed for any medication.

Included mind maps:
- The Life of a Drug in the Body (pharmacokinetics)
- Drug Classifications
- Common Side Effect Categories
- High-Risk Medication Categories
- Drug Schedules (I-V)
- Therapeutic Index & Drug Monitoring
- Common Drug Interactions
- Ways to Memorize Meds

These are perfect for test prep, concept review, and connecting the dots across drug types.

USE THE MEMORY TRICKS & MNEMONICS — TWO

We've included 2 pages of mnemonic "cards" – visual reminders of popular phrases and acronyms students actually use (and remember!).

Cut them out, hang them up, or snap a pic to review on the go.

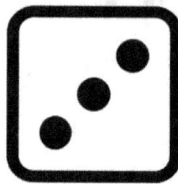

THREE

STUDY WITH PURPOSE

Don't just read — actively study.

As you go through each medication, we encourage you to highlight or underline using this color-coded system to instantly recognize what's what:

- 🟦 Drug Classification & Names
- 🟦 Mechanism of Action
- 🟦 Indications
- 🟦 Side Effects & Adverse Reactions
- 🟦 Nursing Considerations
- Monitoring Requirements
- 🟦 Patient & Caregiver Teaching Points
- ⚫ Black Box Warnings
- Pediatric Considerations
- ⚫ Drug Interactions

(Pro Tip: You don't need 10 highlighters — just make a little color key and underline or box with gel pens or colored pencils!)

COMPLETE THE MIND MAP

FOUR

Once you've highlighted, it's time to organize what you've learned. Use the Medication Mind Map Template in the back of the book to visually break down the drug:

- Class, MOA, Indications
- Side effects, warnings, teaching points
- Your favorite memory trick or mnemonic

This helps you actually process and remember what you just studied — way better than passive reading.

FIVE

TEST WHAT YOU KNOW

After each section, you'll find a QR code that takes you straight to a short NCLEX-style quiz hosted in Google Forms. These aren't just random practice questions — they're carefully crafted to test the most important takeaways from what you just read. But the real magic? <u>The rationales.</u> Whether you get the answer right or wrong, the quiz walks you through the why. Understanding the reasoning behind each answer helps you think like a nurse, not just a test-taker.

It's not about memorizing — it's about making connections, strengthening critical thinking, and applying your knowledge in real clinical scenarios. So take your time, review the rationales, and let them guide you from confusion to clarity.

So don't just read these pages—
interact with them.

📖 Read it. 🎵 Rhyme it. 🧠 Remember it.

> "Nursing is an art: and if it is to be made an art, it requires an exclusive devotion as hard a preparation as any painter's or sculptor's work."
> - Florence Nightingale

PHARMACOLOGY MIND MAPS

COMMON DRUG INTERACTIONS

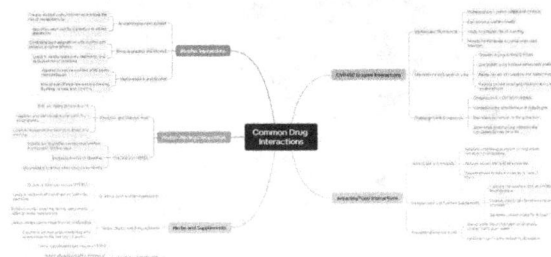

THE LIFE OF A DRUG IN THE BODY

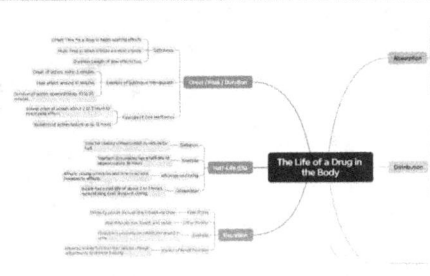
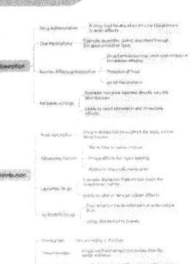

DRUG CLASSIFICATIONS

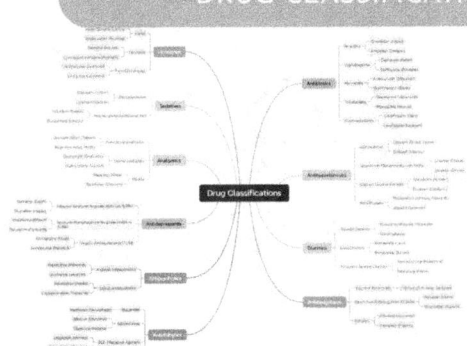

HIGH-RISK MEDICATION CATEGORIES

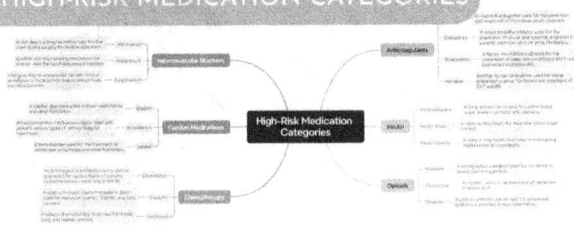

DRUG SCHEDULES

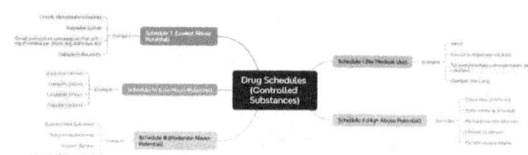

THERAPEUTIC INDEX & DRUG MONITORING

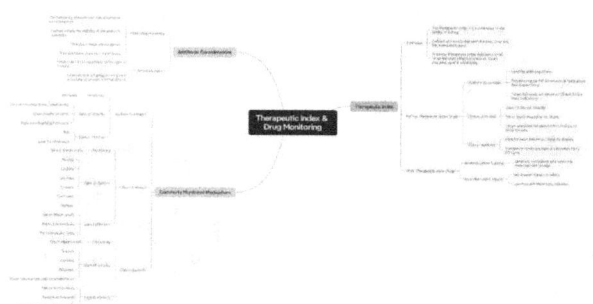

COMMON DRUG INTERACTIONS

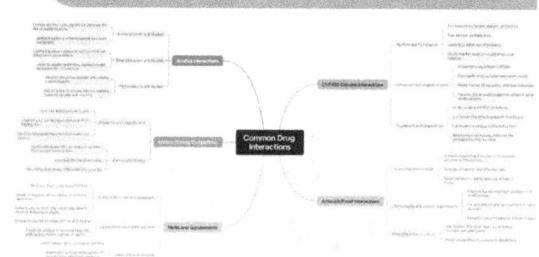

WAYS TO MEMORIZE MEDICATIONS

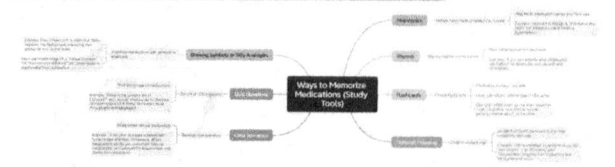

Pharm Mnemonics

SLUDGE
CHOLINERGIC EFFECTS

Salivation, **L**acrimation, **U**rination, **D**iaphoresis, **G**I upset, **E**mesis

Seen in cholinergic overdose or organophosphate poisoning.

ANTICHOLINERGIC
Can't Pee, See, Spit, or Poop

Blurred vision, Urinary retention, Dry mouth, Constipation

Helps recall the hallmark side effects of anticholinergic medications.

NAMES OF INSULINS - L.A.N.D.

Lantus = Long-acting
Apidra = Rapid-acting
Novolog = Rapid-acting
Detemir = Long-acting

BETA-BLOCKERS

"**LOL** Makes the Heart Rate Slow"

All beta-blockers end in "-lol." They decrease heart rate and blood pressure by blocking beta-adrenergic receptors.

ACE INHIBITORS

"**-PRIL** Puts the Pressure Down"

Pressure Reduced In Large vessels. They lower blood pressure by preventing angiotensin II formation.

CALCIUM CHANNEL BLOCKERS

"**V**ery **N**ice **D**rugs"
Verapamil, **N**ifedipine, **D**iltiazem

These drugs dilate blood vessels and slow the heart rate, reducing workload on the heart.

DIURETICS

"**DIM** the Fluid Volume"

Diuretics, **I**ncrease, **M**icturition (urination)

Loop diuretics (e.g., furosemide) or thiazides (e.g., hydrochlorothiazide) help reduce fluid volume, easing edema or hypertension.

ANTICOAGULANTS

"Heparin Works **FAST**, Coumadin **LASTS**"

Heparin is for acute management; Warfarin for long-term prevention. Always monitor lab values (PTT for heparin, PT/INR for warfarin).

ANTIBIOTICS (PENICILLINS & CEPHALOSPORINS)

"Cross Allergy Alerts"

All beta-blockers end in "-lol." They decrease heart rate and blood pressure by blocking beta-adrenergic receptors.

LIDOCAINE TOXICITY

"SAMS"
Slurred speech, **A**ltered central nervous system, **M**uscle twitching, **S**eizures

Recognize signs of lidocaine toxicity.

MEDICATION ADMINISTRATION CHECKLIST

"TRAMP"

Time, **R**oute, **A**mount, **M**edication, **P**atient

Ensure the five rights of medication administration.

EMERGENCY DRUGS TO **"LEAN"** ON

Lidocaine, **E**pinephrine, **A**tropine, **N**aloxone

Common emergency medications administered via endotracheal tube.

Pharm Mnemonics

VENTRICULAR ARRHYTHMIAS
"PALS"
Procainamide, Amiodarone, Lidocaine, Sotalol

Medications used to treat ventricular arrhythmias.

ATRIAL ARRHYTHMIAS
"ABCDE"
Anticoagulants, Beta blockers, Calcium channel blockers, Digoxin, Electrocardioversion

Treatment options for atrial arrhythmias.

MORPHINE SIDE EFFECTS
"MORPHINE"
Miosis, Out of it (sedation), Respiratory depression, Pneumonia (aspiration), Hypotension, Infrequency (constipation, urinary retention), Nausea, Emesis

PARKINSON'S MEDICATIONS
"ALBM"
Amantadine, Levodopa, Bromocriptine, MAO-B inhibitors

Drugs commonly used to manage Parkinson's disease.

THIAZIDES INDICATIONS
"CHIC"
Congestive heart failure, Hypertension, Insipidus (diabetes insipidus), Calcium calculi (kidney stones)

Primary uses for thiazide diuretics.

BRADYCARDIA & HYPOTENSION
"IDEA"
Isoproterenol, Dopamine, Epinephrine, Atropine sulfate

Medications used to manage bradycardia and hypotension.

STEROID SIDE EFFECTS
"6 S's"
Sugar - hyperglycemia, Soggy bones - osteoporosis, Sick - decreased immunity, Sad - depression, Salt - water and salt retention, Sex - decreased libido

LOOP DIURETIC EFFECTS
"LOOP"
Lose sodium, Ototoxicity, Orthostatic hypotension, Potassium loss

Highlights the primary effects and risks of loop diuretics.

ACE INHIBITOR SIDE EFFECTS
"CAPTOPRIL"
Cough, Angioedema, Proteinuria, Taste changes, Orthostatic hypotension, Pregnancy contraindication, Rash, Increased renin, Lower angiotensin II

BETA-BLOCKER CONTRAINDICATIONS
"ABCDE"
Asthma, Block (heart block), COPD, Diabetes mellitus, Electrolyte (hyperkalemia)

Highlights conditions where beta-blockers should be used cautiously or avoided.

GYNECOMASTIA
"DISCO"
Digitalis, Isoniazid, Spironolactone, Cimetidine, Oestrogens

Identifies medications known to cause gynecomastia as a side effect.

TOXICOLOGICAL SEIZURES
"OTIS CAMPBELL"
Organophosphates, Tricyclic antidepressants, Isoniazid, Insulin, Sympathomimetics, Camphor, Cocaine, Amphetamines, Methylxanthines, PCP, Propoxyphene, Phenol, Propranolol, Benzodiazepine withdrawal, Botanicals, Ethanol withdrawal, Lithium, Lidocaine, Lindane, Lead

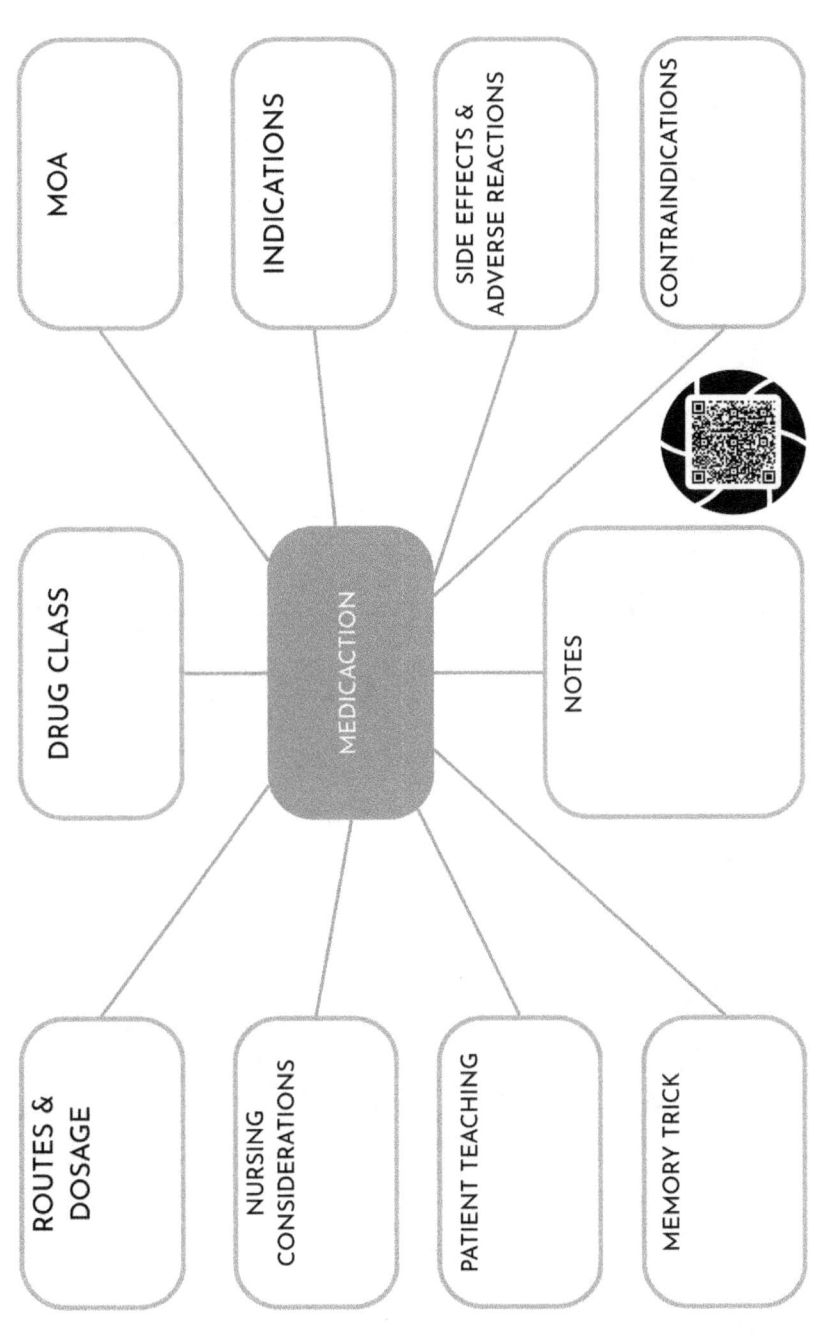

ACETAMINOPHEN (TYLENOL)

Analgesic / Antipyretic

For **fever** high or **aching pain**,
This over-the-counter med is plain.
It blocks the brain's **prostaglandin crew**,
To **lower temp** and **ease pain too**.
Pregnancy-safe? Often yes,
When used with care — not to excess.
In **pregnancy** or **postpartum days**,
It helps with cramps in gentle ways.

But **watch the liver** — that's the key,
Too much can cause **toxicity**.
No more than **4 grams per day**,
Split your doses the **safe-dose way**.
Side effects are **rare but real** —
Rash, **hives**, or **hypersensitivity** feel.
But in **overdose**, you must beware:
Acute liver failure isn't rare.

Check for meds that sneak it in —
"**APAP**" hides in many a bin.
So teach your patient what to do:
Read all labels and see it through.
It's **not an NSAID**, just so you know,
No **anti-inflammatory** power to show.
But **gentle** on the **gut and plate**,
Unlike **NSAIDs** that irritate.

No **Black Box Warning**, but don't be lax —
Caution with alcohol or liver cracks.
Use with **chronic drinkers**? Maybe no —
Monitor **LFTs** if so.

ACYCLOVIR (ZOVIRAX)
Antiviral

For **herpes outbreaks**, this one's key —
It fights the **virus** you can't see.
From **HSV** to **chickenpox**,
It keeps that viral load in a box.
It's a **guanosine analog**, slick and neat,
Stops **viral replication** dead in its beat.
It's not a cure — just slows the tide,
Lessens symptoms you can't hide.

Use in **pregnancy**? Often yes,
For moms with **herpetic distress**.
Helps prevent **neonatal spread**,
When **genital sores** raise fear and dread.
Side effects you might detect:
Nausea, headache, GI upset.
In IV form, here's your clue —
Nephrotoxicity can come through.

So **hydrate well** and **check those labs**,
Renal function's where it stabs.
Monitor **BUN** and **creatinine**,
Keep the kidneys safe and clean.
Teach your patient what it does:
Reduces outbreaks, not because
It's curing — just **controls the flare**,
So **take at onset**, and beware.

It may cause **crystal build-up**, too,
Especially when IV runs through.
So push those **fluids**, flush the line,
Keep that **renal flow** in line.
No **Black Box Warning** here to fear,
But **drug interactions** still appear:
With **probenecid** or **zidovudine**,
Toxicity risks may be seen.

ALBUTEROL (PROAIR, VENTOLIN, PROVENTIL)

Short-Acting Beta-2 Agonist (SABA)

When **bronchospasms** block the way,
This **rescue inhaler** saves the day.
It binds to **beta-2 receptors** tight,
And makes the **airways open** right.
It's used in **asthma** and **COPD**,
And in **pregnancy**, quite safely.
If **wheezing** strikes or **lungs feel tight**,
This med helps patients breathe at night.

Its **mechanism**? Smooth muscle **relax**,
It stops **constriction** in its tracks.
Fast relief — it's quick to act,
But don't rely on it **back-to-back**.
Side effects to teach about:
Tachycardia, **tremor**, and **shaky doubt**.
Some get **palpitations**, feel **anxious too**,
Maybe a **headache** or **nausea brew**.

Monitor HR, especially so
If pregnant patients take it slow.
Too much can lead to **hypokalemia**,
And **high blood sugar** (hyperglycemia).
Teach the **two-puff rule** just right:
Wait 1 minute after the first light.
Rinse the mouth when done the spray,
To keep **dry mouth** and **irritation** away.

There's **no Black Box**, but don't ignore:
If it's **used too often**, it won't restore.
That means their **control is off the track**,
And **long-acting meds** should have their back.
Drug interactions? Yes, take care —
With **beta-blockers**, it's a rough pair.
Add **MAOIs** or **tricyclics** too,
And **toxicity** might break on through

AMOXICILLIN (AMOXIL)
Beta-Lactam Antibiotic (Penicillin Class)

A **broad-spectrum antibiotic** star,
For **bacterial bugs** both near and far.
It binds **bacterial cell wall chains**,
And stops their growth — no more campaigns!
Used in **pregnancy**? Often yes —
For **UTIs**, it's a top success.
Also helps with **strep, ear**, or **throat**,
Or **dental abscess** — worth a note.

Its **mechanism** is crystal clear:
Inhibits **cell wall synthesis** near.
That makes the bug cell **burst and die**,
It's safe for mom and baby, why?
Because it's **Category B**,
With **low fetal risk** in history.
But we still watch for **reactions**, fast —
Like **rash, hives**, or **GI blast**.

Side effects? Not too wild:
Diarrhea, nausea, cramps that riled.
But in **rare allergic states**,
You'll see **anaphylaxis gates**.
So **monitor closely** with the first dose,
Especially if allergy risk is close.
Superinfection may arise —
Like **yeast** or **C. diff** — not a surprise.

Teach to **take it all — don't stop midway**,
Even if symptoms go away.
And **take with food** if tummies churn,
Absorption's fine — they'll slowly learn.
No Black Box Warning, that's a win,
But still take care with **allergies in kin**.
It **interacts with warfarin**, true —
May increase **bleeding risk** in view.

Also with **oral birth control pills**,
It may reduce their **baby-blocking skills**.
So use **back-up birth control**, please —
To prevent surprise pregnancies.

AMOXICILLIN/CLAVULANATE (AUGMENTIN)

Beta-Lactam Antibiotic + Beta-Lactamase Inhibitor

It's **Augmentin** — a **power pair**,
Fighting **bacteria** with extra flair.
Amoxicillin stops **walls from forming**,
While **clavulanate** keeps bugs from swarming.
The **clavulanate** blocks the foes
That make **beta-lactamase enzymes** grow.
So bugs that would resist and win
Get knocked out cold with this strong twin.

Used for **UTIs**, **mastitis**, too,
Or **sinusitis** coming through.
Also great for **post-op wounds**,
And **dental infections** that leave you doomed.
Pregnancy-safe, it's **Category B**,
But still use caution thoughtfully.
Side effects may make a mess —
Diarrhea and **GI distress**.

Some folks get **rash** or **itchy skin**,
And **anaphylaxis** could begin.
So **watch for allergy history**,
Especially **penicillin family**.
Liver function should be watched —
Hepatotoxicity's been notched.
And **superinfections** may arise,
Like **C. diff** or **candida surprise**.

Take with food, it helps digestion,
And lowers GI indigestion.
Teach to **finish the course** — don't quit,
Even if they feel fine a bit.
No Black Box Warning, but here's the deal:
There's still a need to **watch and feel**.

It may **increase warfarin's power**,
So **INR checks** by the hour.

And like with **plain amoxicillin**,
This med can make **birth control** less chillin'.
Use **backup methods** just in case,
To keep surprises from taking place.

AMPICILLIN (PRINCIPEN)
Beta-Lactam Antibiotic (Penicillin Class)

When **Gram-positive bugs** invade,
Or **Listeria** has plans well-laid,
Ampicillin steps to fight,
Blocking cell walls left and right.
Its **mechanism** is clear and smart:
Inhibits **cell wall** from the start.
The **peptidoglycan chains** can't link,
And bacterial strength begins to sink.

Used in **pregnancy** quite a bit —
For **GBS prophylaxis**, it's a hit.
Also treats **chorioamnionitis**,
And helps if **UTIs** persist.
It's **Category B**, so fairly safe,
But watch for **reactions** taking place.
Rash, hives, or in rare conditions,
Anaphylaxis with airway restrictions.

Side effects? Let's make a list:
Nausea, vomiting, GI twist.
May also cause **vaginal yeast**,
When **normal flora** has decreased.
Monitor for allergic signs,
Especially after the first few lines.
If given **IV**, you'll need to check
Renal labs and **liver deck**.

Teach to take it **on empty belly**,
But if there's **nausea**, food is jelly.
Finish the course, don't leave it halfway,
Or bugs might come back another day.

No Black Box Warning, but take note —
Cross-sensitivity gets your vote.
If allergic to **penicillin or cephs**,
They might react — be prepped, not left.

Interacts with oral birth control,
So use **back-up** to stay in control.
And with **allopurinol** on board,
The **rash risk rises**, can't be ignored.

ANASTROZOLE (ARIMIDEX)
Aromatase Inhibitor

When **estrogen feeds** a tumor's flame,
Anastrozole steps in the game.
An **aromatase blocker**, strong and sleek,
It cuts **estrogen** down week by week.
It's used in **postmenopausal care**
For **hormone-positive breast cancer** flare.
By stopping **androgen conversion inside**,
It halts the fuel on which tumors ride.

It **doesn't work** if they're still cycling,
So **only postmenopause** is the right thing.
No **progesterone block** — just E2,
That's **estradiol**, if that's new to you.
Side effects you need to track:
Hot flashes, fatigue, and **aching back**.
Joint pain, weakness, bone loss, too —
So **DEXA scans** are smart to do.

Watch for signs of **fracture risk**,
Especially in the **spine and hip**.
And **cholesterol** may start to rise,
So **lipid panels** would be wise.
Teach to report **vaginal dryness**,
And any **mood swings** or **mental tiredness**.
Take it **daily, same time each day**,
And **don't stop early** unless doc says okay.

There **isn't a Black Box** warning tag,
But still some **risks** can raise a flag:
It may cause **osteoporosis**,
So bone support's a major focus.
Avoid with **tamoxifen** nearby —
They'll **cancel each other**, no lie.
And if she's on **estrogen**, pause —
It defeats **Anastrozole's cause**.

ASPIRIN (LOW-DOSE, 81 MG)
Antiplatelet / NSAID

A tiny dose, but big in might,
This **antiplatelet** aids the fight.
It blocks **COX-1 and COX-2**, see,
To stop **thromboxane A2** activity.
That means less **platelet clumping** near,
Reducing **clots** that moms may fear.
It's used for **cardiac risk control**,
And **preeclampsia prevention** is a key role.

Given in **pregnancy** with care,
Typically from **12 weeks** to prepare.
Especially when there's **risk that's high** —
Like **history of HTN** or **twins nearby**.
Side effects? Let's count a few:
GI upset, and **bleeding**, too.
A **bruise or bleed** can grow quite fast,
Especially if another **NSAID** was passed.

No big dose for OB care —
High-dose aspirin? Moms beware.
That can harm the **ductus** flow,
And **bleed the fetus** — risk to know.
Teach your patient: **take with food**,
It helps prevent a **GI feud**.
Don't crush **enteric-coated pills**,
And skip if they've had **bleeding ills**.

Monitor platelets, check for signs
Of **bleeding gums** or **blood in lines**.
Teach to report **ringing in ears**,
It may mean **toxicity nears**.

There's **no Black Box Warning** for the low,
But still, **precaution** is the way to go.
And avoid with **NSAIDs**, **warfarin**,
Or **herbals** like **ginkgo** thrown in.

ATENOLOL (TENORMIN)
Beta-1 Selective Blocker

When the heart beats fast or high,
Atenolol can help it lie.
It blocks the **beta-1 receptor**,
To slow the pace and make it better.
It's used for **HTN, angina**, too,
And sometimes for a **pregnancy** crew.
But caution here — let's be precise,
The risks can come with a fetal price.

It **reduces HR and BP**,
Decreasing **cardiac workload** carefully.
But crosses through the **placental gate**,
Which means we must evaluate.
Side effects can make things rough:
Bradycardia, fatigue, and **cough**.
Some get **dizzy, cold,** or **blue**,
From **peripheral vasoconstriction**, too.

In pregnancy, risks include:
Fetal growth restriction (not so good).
Low birth weight and **bradycardia**,
So **monitor that baby's area**.
Teach to **never stop abruptly**,
It could spike BP quite disruptly.
Take it **daily**, same time best —
And monitor during **rest and stress**.

Watch for signs of **hypoglycemia**,
It may **mask** it — that's academia!
So if she's **diabetic**, use great care —
Low sugar signs may not be there.
No **Black Box Warning**, but still take note:
Abrupt withdrawal gets our vote
For danger signs — so we taper slow,
And educate before they go.

It **interacts with other meds**
That drop the **heart rate**, clear as threads.
Like **calcium channel blockers**, be aware —
Or **digoxin**, with double care.

AZITHROMYCIN (ZITHROMAX)

Macrolide Antibiotic

For **chlamydia**, **cervicitis**, too,
Azithromycin comes to you.
It stops the bugs from making chains —
By blocking **protein synth domains**.
It binds the **50S ribosome**,
So **bacterial growth** can't find a home.
It's **broad-spectrum**, works quite fast,
With a **long half-life** that makes it last.

In **pregnancy**, it's often picked,
For **STIs** that must be licked.
One big dose is all it takes —
A **Z-Pak** clears those micro fakes.
Side effects? A few to know:
Nausea, vomiting, GI woe.
QT prolongation, rare but true —
So watch the **EKG** if they're high-risk, too.

Liver toxicity may appear,
So monitor **LFTs** once a year.
Teach to **avoid antacids** close,
They bind the drug and make it gross.
Take it **with or without some food**,
But **don't skip doses** — that's just rude.
And finish off the full Z-course,
To stop resistance at the source.

No **Black Box Warning**, but beware
Of **cardiac risks** in those with care.
Older adults and **heart conditions**
May need some closer **monitoring missions**.
It **interacts** with **warfarin**, too —
Increasing **bleeding risk** for you.
And with **QT drugs**, double-check —
Like **amiodarone** or **haloperidol**, heck!

BENZOCAINE (AMERICAINE, DERMOPLAST)

Local Anesthetic (Ester Type)

For **numbing pain** on skin or gum,
Benzocaine can make things numb.
It **blocks sodium channels** in the nerves,
So pain signals don't get on your nerves.
It's used for **episiotomy tears**,
Or **hemorrhoid pain** in postpartum care.
Also found in **lozenges, gels,** and **sprays**,
To soothe **oral sores** or **toothache days**.

Topical only, that's the rule —
Never inject it — that's not cool.
Apply in **small amounts**, not wide,
And **wash your hands** when you've applied.
Side effects are pretty rare,
But **skin reactions** may occur there.
Itching, burning, or **red skin tone**,
Should make you stop — leave it alone.

More severe (though seldom seen):
Methemoglobinemia on the scene.
It turns the blood a **bluish hue**,
And lowers **oxygen** getting through.
So **don't use on broken skin** or sore,
And never apply **more and more**.
Especially not near **infant gums**,
For teething pain — that rule still runs.

No **Black Box Warning**, but the FDA
Warns **infants** could see danger that way.
So **avoid in children under two**,
Unless your provider tells you to.
No major **interactions**, yay!
But still use caution every day.
Especially when using **other numbing gels**,
To avoid **toxic overlapping spells**.

BUPROPION (WELLBUTRIN, ZYBAN)
Atypical Antidepressant / Smoking Cessation Aid

When **depression clouds the mind**,
And **energy** is hard to find,
Bupropion can lift that fog,
Without the **weight gain** or **libido clog**.
It **inhibits reuptake** — dopamine,
And **norepinephrine** — nice and clean.
But not **serotonin**, unlike the rest,
So it helps with **focus, drive**, and zest.
Branded **Wellbutrin** for low mood,
And **Zyban** if you're quitting food...
(Just kidding — that's **nicotine**),
But yes, it helps you ditch that scene.
It's often used in **postpartum blues**,
Or **perinatal** mental health news.
But **pregnancy risk**? That's debated —
The research still is **complicated**.
Side effects may stir the pot:
Dry mouth, sweating, insomnia — a lot.
Some get **anxiety, headache pain**,
And **weight loss**, if that's your gain.
But here's the kicker: **seizure risk** —
Especially when doses get brisk.
So don't exceed the **400 mg/day**,
Or 450 if they say okay.
Black Box Warning leads the chart:
For **suicidal thoughts** in youth — take heart.
So screen for risks in **pediatrics**,
And **perinatal patients** with mood erratics.
Don't give it if they're **anorexic**,
Or have a **seizure disorder** — that's too risky.

Same for those who've had **alcohol withdrawal**,
Or **benzo tapers** — not safe at all.
Drug interactions you should know:
With **MAOIs**, it's a hard no-go.
Also watch for **CYP2B6** plays,
Like **ritonavir** and some protease.
Teach to **take it early**, not at night,
Since **insomnia** may take flight.
And if they miss a dose or two?
Don't double up — that won't do.

CALCIUM CARBONATE (TUMS, CALTRATE)

Calcium Supplement / Antacid

For **bones** and **baby**, this one's gold,
Calcium carbonate helps you hold.
It treats **heartburn** and **acid pain**,
And builds strong bones again and again.
It works by **neutralizing acid** flow,
In the **stomach** where discomfort grows.
Also boosts your **calcium stores**,
To fight off **osteoporosis wars**.

In **pregnancy**, it's often used
When heartburn leaves the gut confused.
Plus baby needs those **minerals strong** —
So calcium's a lifelong song.
Side effects? They're mild, you see:
Constipation, and **bloating spree**.
And if you take it **way too much**,
You risk a **calcium overload touch**.

Too much can cause **kidney stones**,
Or throw off other **electrolyte zones**.
So don't go popping them like candy —
Even though the taste is handy.
Teach your patient not to mix
With **iron**, or they won't absorb the fix.
It also blocks some **meds and pills**,
Like **tetracyclines** and **thyroid fills**.

Take it **separately** by an hour or two,
From other meds they're working through.

And **with food** is best for bone support —
That's how it's absorbed, research reports.
No Black Box Warning, but still say:
Avoid with **severe kidney decay**.
Check **phosphorus** and **renal labs**,
If their kidney function drags.

CARBETOCIN (DURATOCIN)
Uterotonic Agent

A **uterotonic** strong and swift, To give the **uterus** one last lift. It helps prevent a **bleeding tide**, Once birth has brought the babe outside.
It mimics **oxytocin's** way, To keep **postpartum hemorrhage** at bay. By binding to those muscle sites, It starts those **contraction-driven fights**.
Used right after **vaginal birth**, Or C-section's return to earth— To stop the blood from flowing free, It clamps the womb's **vasculature tree**.
Avoid in cases where it's known That **hypertension's seeds are sown**. Or if the mom has heart disease, You'll skip this drug and look for ease.
Most side effects are rather mild, Like **nausea**, seen in mom and child. Some may feel **a flushing face**, Or tremble in a brief, strange place.
But rare events deserve our eye— Like **chest pain**, or a **BP** high. Watch for **bronchospasm**, though it's slight, And **anaphylaxis**—worst of fright.
Check **vitals** first—**especially BP**, And keep that **oxygen tank** handy. Observe the **fundus**, firm and tight, And **lochia flow** throughout the night.
Don't give with other **uterotonics**, Or drugs that have **vasoconstricting tonics**. Space your meds with practiced care, To avoid a **vascular nightmare**.
Teach your patient what to feel— Some **cramping** as the uterus heals. Reassure and help her rest, And monitor her **bleeding test**.
Though **no black box** warning here exists, The nurse must still be **on the list** To **monitor reactions** and explain What's happening post-placental strain.
So **Carbetocin**, one clear dose, Stands guard where danger's often close. A final push to clamp and bind, And keep the **mother's strength aligned**.

CARBOPROST TROMETHAMINE (HEMABATE)

Prostaglandin Analog (Oxytocic Agent)

When **postpartum bleeding** won't quit fast,
Carboprost helps make it last.
It mimics **prostaglandin F2-alpha**,
To make the **uterine tone** snap back at ya.
It causes **uterine contractions tight**,
To stop that bleed and make things right.
Used for **PPH (postpartum hemorrhage)** now,
When **oxytocin** just won't wow.

It's also used in **2nd trimester**
To induce abortion when it must occur.
But in OB, it's best known still
For **controlling bleeding** with serious skill.
Side effects — oh, quite a few:
Nausea, vomiting, diarrhea, too.
May cause **fever, flushing, chills**,
And **bronchospasm** — that gives us thrills (not really).

Contraindications? Here's the key:
Asthma, renal, and **hepatic disease**.
Also avoid with **PID**,
Or in moms with **heart disease** history.
Monitor vitals with each dose,
Especially when **BP** goes close.
Check for **bleeding, uterine tone**,
And if they're **breathing** on their own.

Teach they may have **cramping pain**,
And flu-like symptoms in their frame.
But reassure — it's short and done,
The goal is saving everyone.
No Black Box Warning, but use with care
In **respiratory-compromised** moms out there.
And if combined with **other uterotonics**,
The **uterus** may go supersonic.

CEFOTAXIME (CLAFORAN)
3rd Generation Cephalosporin (Beta-Lactam Antibiotic)

When **infection hits** and stakes are high,
Cefotaxime is standing by.
A **broad-spectrum cephalosporin** third,
It fights off bugs both tough and absurd.
It blocks **cell wall synthesis** in place,
So bacteria lose their outer space.
Works on **Gram-negatives**, tough to beat,
And still gets **Gram-positives** in retreat.

Used for **intrapartum fever** signs,
Or **chorioamnionitis** lines.
Also key for **neonatal sepsis**,
When baby's system needs defenses.
Side effects you should expect:
Diarrhea, rash, and **GI upset**.
May cause **eosinophilia**,
Or **superinfections** like **C. diff area**.

If given **IV**, don't miss the cue:
Watch for **phlebitis** at the view.
And **renal function** must be seen,
Especially if the mom's not keen.
Teach that it's a **hospital drug**,
Not one you take with just a mug.
Usually given **in the vein**,
To treat infection deep in the brain
(like meningitis!).

No Black Box Warning, but here's the scoop:

Can alter **gut flora** and baby's poop.
In neonates, use with thought,
To avoid **bilirubin battles** they fought.
Watch **BUN, creatinine,** and signs
Of **liver stress** or **platelet declines**.
Check for **hypersensitivity**,
Especially with **penicillin history**.

Also note: with **live vaccines**,
You'll want to wait to keep it clean.
And with **diuretics**, be aware —
Nephrotoxicity risk is there.

CEFOTETAN (CEFOTAN)
2nd Generation Cephalosporin (Beta-Lactam Antibiotic)

When **C-sections** bring infection's threat,
Cefotetan says, "Not just yet!"
It stops **cell wall construction** cold,
So **bacteria die**, their structure rolled.
It's a **2nd gen cephalosporin** drug,
That battles **aerobes, anaerobes**, snug.
Used for **surgical prophylaxis**,
Especially in **OB/GYN practice**.

It's perfect for **pelvic procedures**,
Or **postpartum uterine fevers**.
Great for **pre-op dosing**, clear and bold,
To stop **Gram-negative bugs** from taking hold.
Side effects may still appear:
Nausea, vomiting, diarrhea near.
And **rash, itching**, or **fever chills**,
Can show if the body's had its fill.

It may prolong the **PT** or **INR**,
So with **anticoagulants**, don't go far.
And like most **beta-lactam crew**,
It may bring **C. diff colitis** through.
Watch for **bleeding risk** with care,
Especially if they're **low on K** in there.
It also may cause **disulfiram-like pain**,
If **alcohol** enters the vein.

No Black Box Warning, but still assess

For **renal function** and **GI distress**.
Use **caution with penicillin allergy**,
They may cross-react unexpectedly.
Monitor labs for any decline —
Especially **CBC**, and **creatinine line**.
And if used before a **C-section cut**,
Give **within 60 minutes** — clean and shut!

CEFTRIAXONE (ROCEPHIN)
3rd Generation Cephalosporin (Beta-Lactam Antibiotic)

Ceftriaxone, strong and sleek,
Fights off bugs both bold and bleak.
A **broad-spectrum IV/IM** shot,
It works where weaker drugs do not.
It stops the **cell wall** from building tall,
So **bacteria burst** — no wall at all.
Works great on **Gram-negative strains**,
And **STIs** causing pelvic pains.

Used for **gonorrhea** first in line,
And for **PID**, it works just fine.
Also used for **chorio**,
And **post-op fever** if it shows.
In **pregnancy**, it's **Category B**,
But **not for neonates**, typically —
It displaces **bilirubin** fast,
Risking **kernicterus** that can last.

Side effects? A short review:
Diarrhea, **rash**, and maybe **flu**.
Injection site pain is pretty real,
And **phlebitis** may steal the deal.
It can also cause **gallbladder sludge**,
So **LFTs** are good to judge.
And if they've got a **penicillin past**,
A **cross-reaction** risk may last.

Teach it's given **once a day**,
A powerful dose that holds its sway.
Dilute if IV, slow the rate,
To minimize discomfort at the gate.
No Black Box Warning, but hold tight

If they've had **severe liver fights**.
And don't mix with **calcium IV**,
In **neonates**, that's risky, see?

Drug interactions? Just a few:
It may **enhance warfarin's view**,
So monitor for **bleeding signs**,
And **platelet counts** in tough decline.

CEPHALEXIN (KEFLEX)
1st Generation Cephalosporin (Beta-Lactam Antibiotic)

When **bacteria** start their fight,
Cephalexin brings the light.
It stops their **cell wall** piece by piece,
So infections shrink and symptoms cease.
Used for **UTIs**, and **skin that's red**,
And **mastitis** when the breast is fed.
It's **Category B**, so often picked
When a **pregnant mom** is getting sick.

It's **oral only**, not IV,
And fights off bugs in **soft tissue** and **pee**.
It works on many **Gram-positives**, too,
But **Gram-negatives**? Just a few.
Side effects? A minor list:
GI upset, and **rash on wrists**.
Some may feel a bit **fatigued**,
And rare **allergies** may be intrigued.

If allergic to **penicillin's line**,
They may have a **cross-reaction** sign.
So ask before the first dose starts,
And check for **itching**, **hives**, or **hearts** (racing!).
Teach to **take with food** if queasy,
And complete the course — don't get lazy.
Skipping pills can breed resistance,
And make bugs grow with persistence.

No Black Box Warning, but still assess
For **kidney issues** or GI distress.
Watch for signs of **superinfection**,
Like **yeast** or **C. diff** recollection.
Drug interactions? Not a ton —
But can enhance **warfarin** (bleeding fun).
Check **INR** if they're on both,
To keep that **clotting** under oath.

CETIRIZINE (ZYRTEC)
2nd Generation Antihistamine (H1 Blocker)

When **allergies** bring itchy doom,
Cetirizine clears up the room.
It blocks **histamine at H1 sites**,
So you can breathe and sleep at night.
Used for **rhinitis, hives, allergic flare**,
And safe for **pregnant moms** with care.
It's **Category B**, so it's well-known
For being **safer** than the older zone.

It doesn't cause as much **drowsy fog**
Like **diphenhydramine** or that log.
Still, some folks feel a little slow,
So caution if they **drive or go**.
Side effects are mild and few:
Dry mouth, fatigue, or feeling "blue."
Some get **headaches**, rarely worse,
But nothing wild for this small verse.

Monitor for relief of signs —
Less **itching, sneezing, watery lines**.
Check if **symptoms improve** in days,
Or if they need to switch the ways.
Teach to **take it once per day**,
With or without food's okay.
Don't mix with **alcohol or dope**,
It adds to drowsy's slippery slope.

No Black Box Warning here,
But still be wise and crystal clear:
In **renal disease**, adjust the dose —
It's cleared by **kidneys** more than most.

It's got few **interactions** true,
But stacking **CNS depressants**? Boo.
So don't mix in too many meds
That **slow the brain** or **weigh your head**.

CITALOPRAM (CELEXA)
Selective Serotonin Reuptake Inhibitor (SSRI)

An **SSRI**, calm and clear, For **depression**, **panic**, **mood**, and fear. It lifts the lows, the mind rewires, And **raises serotonin's** fires.
Its name is **Citalopram**, true— With brand-name **Celexa** known to you. It **blocks reuptake** in the brain, So more **serotonin** can remain.
Prescribed for **MDD**, no doubt, And sometimes **anxiety's** drawn-out bout. It helps with **OCD** as well, Where looping thoughts and habits dwell.
But use it not in **MAOI** ties, Or **QT prolongation** risks arise. Avoid with meds that **raise the QT**, Or when **liver function** fails to be.
Watch **nausea**, **fatigue**, and **dry mouth**, too, And **sweating** more than most would do. **Drowsiness**, or feeling flat— But these effects may fade off at that.
A rarer few may feel the sting Of **serotonin syndrome's** ring— With **fever**, **tremors**, and **confused mind**, A **life-threatening state** of chemical grind.
Before you start, check **EKG**, And monitor **heart rhythm carefully**. **Electrolytes** may play a part— Like **low potassium** or **magnesium's heart**.
Teach patients not to **suddenly quit**, Or **discontinuation symptoms** may hit: **Dizziness**, **zaps**, or a **rushing mind**— Withdraw it slow and be aligned.

Advise to watch for **worsening mood**, Or thoughts that darkly may intrude. **Suicidal signs** must be addressed, Especially when new meds are pressed.
Takes weeks before they feel it grow, Improvement comes so **very slow**. So tell them not to toss the pack— Their light is coming, bring it back.
Pregnancy use—assess the risk, Though safer than some older lists. But **lactation** could pass it through, So weigh what's safest for baby too. There's **no black box** for no good cause— Its warning gives the nurse a pause. Watch for **suicide**, age defined— Especially for the **younger mind**.
Citalopram, a helpful tool, But one that must be used with rule. A gentle hand, a nurse's eye— Can guard the brain while lifting sky.

CLINDAMYCIN (CLEOCIN)
Lincosamide Antibiotic

When **penicillin's out the door**,
Clindamycin brings back the war.
It blocks **protein synthesis** with grace,
At the **50S ribosome** site, in place.
It's used in OB for lots of things:
Bacterial vaginosis, uterine flings,
Chorioamnionitis, wound site care,
And **GBS** when **penicillin's a scare.**

It hits **Gram-positive** bugs just fine,
And **anaerobes** down the pelvic line.
Great for **dental, skin,** or **vaginal gunk,**
When infections start to feel sunk.
Side effects? The biggest fear:
⚠ **C. diff colitis** — loud and clear.
So if there's **diarrhea, stomach pain,**
Test for **toxins** in the strain.

Also causes **nausea, rash, metallic taste,**
And **elevated LFTs** in haste.
Injection pain or **phlebitis**, true,
If you're giving it **IV through and through.**
No Black Box for most conditions —
But for **C. diff**, it gets admissions.
Warn the patient of that sign,
And hydrate well if symptoms align.

Monitor the gut and **bowel flow,**
Especially if taken long in a row.
And if the mom is breastfeeding?
Watch for **yeast,** or **GI misleading.**

Teach to take it **with full water,**
And **space from antacids** like you oughta.
Finish the course, don't quit the pack,
Even if those symptoms pull back.

Interactions? Just a few:
With **neuromuscular blockers**, it might skew.
So in labor with **Mag sulfate drip,**
Be sure you're watching that muscle grip.

CLOMIPHENE CITRATE (CLOMID, SEROPHENE)
Selective Estrogen Receptor Modulator (SERM)

When **ovulation** takes a pause,
Clomiphene steps in with applause.
It tricks the brain with **estrogen lies**,
So **FSH** and **LH** can rise.
That rise then wakes the **ovary's spark**,
To **release an egg** and hit the mark.
It's the first step in **fertility care**,
For **PCOS** or cycles rare.

It binds **estrogen receptors** tight,
In the **hypothalamus**, day or night.
That makes the body think there's low supply,
So it boosts the **hormones** way up high.
Taken orally, once a day,
For **5 days**, then wait and pray.
Usually started on **day 3 or 5**,
To help those follicles grow and thrive.

Side effects are real — don't gloss:
Hot flashes, bloating, nausea, loss
Of patience from the **mood swings wild**,
And **headache** feelings not so mild.
Rarely comes a bigger scare:
⚠ **Ovarian hyperstimulation** — beware.
Pelvic pain, swelling, weight that spikes,
Call the doctor — don't roll the dice.

Also note the **twin risk's true**,
It may make **more than one egg** too.

So teach about the **multiple chance**,
When they plan that baby dance.
No **Black Box Warning**, but keep in mind:
Avoid in **hepatic disease of any kind**,
And **uterine bleeding** that's not explained —
Or **ovarian cysts** that are inflamed.

Monitor ovulation signs,
Ultrasounds, and **hormone lines**.
And teach: "This med's just step one,"
Success may need more cycles run.

CLOTRIMAZOLE (LOTRIMIN, MYCELEX, GYNE-LOTRIMIN)

When **yeast** begins to itch and burn,
Clotrimazole helps the tide turn.
It stops the **fungal cell wall's build**,
So **candida's army** gets quietly killed.
It **inhibits ergosterol** deep inside,
Breaking down the **fungal wall's pride**.
Used for **vaginal infections** the most,
It can also treat **athlete's foot** and **toes that roast**.

In OB, it's often picked,
For **pregnant patients** who've been nicked
By yeast from **hormonal shifts or meds**,
Or lingering infections after birth beds.
Topical or vaginal forms are best,
With **suppositories**, **creams**, or **1%**.
Safe in **pregnancy**, often **preferred**,
Over oral meds, where risks are stirred.

Side effects? Mostly mild:
Itching, **burning**, or **vaginal wild**.
A little **cramping** or **red skin sting**,
But rarely more than a passing thing.
Teach: apply it **at bedtime slow**,
So it stays in place, not on the go.

Wear **cotton undies**, skip the thong,
And **no douching** while the meds are strong.

No **Black Box Warning** here to fear,
But still, use care if **symptoms reappear**.
If **no relief in 7 days**,
A **follow-up** should guide the phase.
Little **systemic absorption** is done,
So **drug interactions**? Usually none.
But if also using **vaginal meds**,
Space them out — don't mix those threads.

CODEINE/ACETAMINOPHEN (TYLENOL #3, #4)

Opioid + Analgesic Combo

When **postpartum pain** won't let go,
This **combo med** can ease the blow.
Acetaminophen brings the heat down low,
While **codeine** tells the pain to go.
Codeine is an **opioid light**,
That binds to **mu receptors** tight.
It dulls the brain's **pain perception**,
While **acetaminophen** adds protection.

Used for **episiotomy pain**,
Or **after C-section aches remain**.
But caution is the nurse's friend —
Because **breastfeeding risks** extend.
Side effects? You'll want to teach:
Drowsiness, nausea, constipation breach.
Dizziness, dry mouth, GI distress,
And **respiratory depression**, nonetheless.

Black Box Warning loud and clear:
For **ultra-rapid metabolizers** — steer clear!
Some convert **codeine to morphine** fast,
Which can harm the **infant** — effects may last.
So in **lactating moms**, take pause,
This med may break **safety laws**.
Assess if safer options lie,
Before giving **Tylenol with an opioid tie**.

Monitor pain, and **respiratory rate**,
Check for **sedation** and signs too late.
Bowel function should be assessed,
And offer **fluids, fiber, walking rest**.
Teach to avoid **alcohol swigs**,
And **driving** until they're off the meds' gigs.
Don't double-dose with other "Tylenol" names —
That's how **liver failure** claims.

Drug interactions you should screen:
With **CNS depressants** — that's not clean.
Also watch with **MAOIs**,
Or **sedative meds** that slow the highs.

COMBINED ORAL CONTRACEPTIVES (COCS)

Estrogen + Progestin Hormonal Contraceptive

A daily pill, with powerful flair,
COCs are birth control with care.
They combine **estrogen** and **progestin**,
To stop ovulation from within.
They **suppress LH and FSH**,
So the **egg stays put** inside its cage.
They **thicken cervical mucus** too,
So sperm can't swim their way on through.
Used for more than just control —
They help with **acne**, **cramps**, and **cycle goals**.
Treat **PCOS**, and **endometriosis** pain,
And **lighten flow** when periods drain.
But there are **risks** that must be known,
So nurses teach before they're shown:
Side effects? A long list here:
Nausea, **headaches**, and **mood swings** near.
Breast tenderness, **spotting** days,
And sometimes **weight** in subtle ways.
Black Box Warning stands tall —
For **smokers over 35**, most of all.
The risk of **clots**, **stroke**, or **MI**
Can rise and hit the heart and sky.
So screen for **DVT signs** quick —
Leg pain, vision changes, chest that's thick.
And teach them when to **seek the doc**,
If warning signs begin to knock.

Contraindications? Quite a few:
Like **hypertension**, and **liver, too**.
Migraines with aura, and **history of clots**,
Or **breast cancer** risks connect the dots.
Teach to take the pill same time,
Every day — stay in line.
If they **miss one**, it's no big deal —
But **three missed pills**? That's a slippery feel.
Teach to **use condoms** for a week,
If **starting late** or **safety's weak**.
And **antibiotics**, like **rifampin**, may
Reduce the pill's effect that day.

CONJUGATED ESTROGENS (PREMARIN)

Estrogen Hormone Replacement

When **estrogen** is low or gone,
Premarin helps to carry on.
It's **conjugated estrogens** from mares,
Restoring balance with hormone flares.
It treats **hot flashes, vaginal dry**,
And mood swings that can make one cry.
Used in **menopause** and **surgical loss**,
When ovaries are gone — or on pause.

It works by **binding estrogen sites**,
To bring those hormone levels right.
Improves **bone density, mood**, and **skin**,
And keeps the **urogenital tissues in**.
But ⚠ **risks** are real and bold and loud —
So **careful screening** is allowed.
Blood clots, stroke, or **breast cancer rise** —
So weigh the benefits and size.

Black Box Warnings, let's review:
→ For **endometrial cancer** too.
→ For **cardiovascular events** in age —
Especially past the **menopause stage**.
→ And when used without **progestin**,
In **intact uterus**, risk sets in.

Side effects? Here's the spread:
Breast pain, nausea, and **spotting red**.
Bloating, headaches, and **mood swings** hit,
And sometimes **weight** will slowly flit.
Monitor with yearly exams —
Mammograms, and **pelvic scans**.
Teach about **DVT signs**, too —
Leg pain, vision change, or **chest that's blue**.

It's **contraindicated** in:
→ **Active clotting**, or if they've been
→ Through **estrogen-related cancer**,
→ Or have **liver disease** — don't chance her.
Teach to **use the lowest dose**,
For the **shortest time** — that's the most.
And always review **other hormone meds**,
To avoid double **estrogen threads**.

COPPER IUD (PARAGARD)
Non-Hormonal Long-Acting Reversible Contraceptive (LARC)

No **hormones** here, just **copper pride**,
This IUD works from inside.
It's placed within the **uterine wall**,
And stops the sperm from swimming at all.
It creates **inflammation local**,
Making sperm survival not so vocal.
The **copper ions** make them fail,
So **fertilization** derails.

It lasts for up to **ten full years**,
No daily pills, no monthly fears.
It's also used in **emergency**,
Placed within **five days** effectively.
Side effects include some things:
Heavier bleeding, cramping stings,
Spotting in the first few months,
And maybe some **menstrual bumps**.

It may cause **uterine expulsion**,
Or rarely, **pelvic wall intrusion**.
PID is a slight concern,
If **STIs** are left to burn.
There's **no Black Box Warning** here,
But still, use judgment crystal clear.
Screen for **pregnancy** before you start,
And **check for strings** once they depart.

It's **contraindicated** when:
They have **active pelvic infection** then,
Or **unexplained uterine bleeding** persists,
Or they have **Wilson's disease** on their list.

Teach patients how to **feel the strings**,
To know the device is doing its thing.
And if the strings seem lost or gone,
They should follow up before too long.

DESOGESTREL
Progestin (Synthetic Progesterone)

A **progestin** pill with steady aim,
Desogestrel plays the birth control game.
It **thickens cervical mucus** walls,
And sometimes **blocks ovulation calls**.
In **combo pills**, it's paired just right
With **ethinyl estradiol** in sight.
But it also comes as a **POP**,
For those who can't take **estrogen's drop**.

It's safe in **breastfeeding** postpartum, too,
When **estrogen** is not the best to do.
Also helps with **painful periods**,
And cuts down **acne** flare-up surges.
Side effects? You may observe:
Irregular bleeding, or **no bleeding curve**.
Some feel **headaches**, **breast tenderness**,
Or **mood shifts** with some edginess.

There's **no Black Box Warning** on its own,
But **combo pills** with it have shown
Increased clot risk — that's the line
When **estrogen** and **smoking** intertwine.
Contraindications still apply:
Breast cancer, **liver disease**, or **clot risk high**.
And for those with **undiagnosed bleed**,
A full workup is the need.

Teach to take it **same time each day**,
Even a **3-hour delay** may sway.
If they miss, use **backup** quick —
The **window for error** is very slick.
There are few **interactions** in the mix,
But **enzyme inducers** may play tricks.
So with **anticonvulsants** or **St. John's Wort**,
Efficacy may come up short.

DEXAMETHASONE (DECADRON)

Glucocorticoid / Corticosteroid

A **steroid** with a mighty name, **Dexamethasone** plays many a game. From swelling, rash, and asthma's fire, To **preterm lungs** it can inspire.
Known as **Decadron**, it stands tall, A **glucocorticoid** that does it all. It dampens **inflammation's** spark, And **immune response** that grows too dark.
It's given **oral**, **IV**, or **IM**, Depending on the patient's plan. And often used before **week thirty-four**, To help the lungs in **babies born before**.
Indications? Quite a range: **Allergic states**, and those quite strange. **Cerebral edema**, **shock**, or **flare**— Even **COVID protocols** now care.
But use with caution, never light, In **infections** hidden out of sight. Avoid with **fungal illness deep**, Or when **live vaccines** still must sleep.
Side effects may come in waves— **Insomnia**, or **mood that caves**. **Hyperglycemia**, **GI pain**, And sometimes **weight the cheeks** may gain.
More severe is **Cushing's face**, With **buffalo hump** and moon-round grace. Or **osteoporosis** in long use, Where **fragile bones** may come loose.
Check **glucose**, **weight**, and **BP high**, And watch the **WBC** multiply. Check for **hypokalemia's signs**, And **infection** hiding in the lines.
Taper slowly—don't just quit, Or **adrenal crisis** may then hit. The body's made to lean on this, So wean it down, don't go amiss.
Teach your patient not to stop, To take it with **food**, not as a drop. Report **black stools**, or **vision's haze**, Or **wounds that take too many days**.
No **black box warning** comes in tow, But every nurse must surely know: It masks **infection**, changes labs, And slows down **healing's** post-op grabs.
So **Dexamethasone**, strong and wide, A steroid used on many sides. With power comes the need to guide— A careful dose, a nurse beside.

DICLOFENAC (VOLTAREN, CATAFLAM)
Nonsteroidal Anti-Inflammatory Drug (NSAID)

When **cramps** or **inflammation** rise,
Diclofenac is your ally wise.
It blocks **COX enzymes**, stops **prostaglandins**,
And helps ease pain with steady hands.
Used for **dysmenorrhea pain**,
Or **post-op aches** that still remain.
Also helps with **pelvic strain**,
From **endometriosis** or **joint pain**.

Side effects may soon appear:
GI upset, or **ulcers near**.
Nausea, heartburn, headache too,
And **edema** in a swollen shoe.
Black Box Warnings to review:
Risk of **cardiovascular events** is true.
Like **stroke, MI**, especially when
Used long-term or with heart-risk men.

There's also risk of **GI bleeds**,
Like **ulcers, perfs**, and **gut wall needs**.
So monitor for **bloody stools**,
And teach patients NSAID rules.
Use **caution in pregnancy**, especially late,
In **third trimester**, it's not great.
It may cause **premature ductus close**,
So avoid past **30 weeks** — that's known.

Contraindications you should scan:
Peptic ulcer, kidney plan,
Severe liver disease, or **heart attack**
Are reasons to hold **Diclofenac**.
Teach to take it **with some food**,
To guard the gut and lift the mood.
Avoid with **alcohol or aspirin** pairs,
And **watch the BP** — it flares in there.

Drug interactions may include:
Anticoagulants, NSAID feud.
ACE inhibitors, lithium, too —
Can cause levels to skew through.

DINOPROSTONE (CERVIDIL, PREPIDIL, PROSTIN E2)

Prostaglandin E2 Analog (Oxytocic Agent)

When **labor's near** but **cervix tight**,
Dinoprostone helps it ripen right.
A **prostaglandin** smooth and wise,
It softens, thins, and dilates size.
Placed **vaginally** in gel or tab,
Or as a **retractable insert slab**.
It **stimulates contractions**, too,
Helping baby **break on through**.

Used for **induction, late-term care**,
Or **fetal demise** when it's there.
Also used for **missed miscarriage**,
To help the body take the carriage.
Side effects can start to show:
Nausea, vomiting, fever glow.
Some feel **back pain, chills**, or **cramps**,
As **uterine tone** amps up like amps.

⚠ **Monitor closely** after start —
Watch **FHR** and **contraction chart**.
It may cause **uterine hyperstim**,
Which can put **baby at fetal risk** grim.
⚠ **Contraindicated** when:
There's **non-reassuring fetal pattern** then,
Or **previous uterine surgery**,
Like **classical C-sections** — that's a key.

There is **no Black Box Warning** tag,
But still, be sharp and never lag.
Monitor vitals, assess **pain and tone**,
And **remove insert** if risks are shown.

Teach it may cause **pelvic pain**,
And sometimes **diarrhea in the chain**.
Let them know to **lay back down**,
For **2 hours** post-insertion round.

Watch for **tachysystole** signs —
More than 5 contractions in 10-minute lines.
Have **terbutaline** standing near,
In case the uterus shifts to gear.

DIPHENHYDRAMINE (BENADRYL)

1st Generation Antihistamine (H1 Blocker)

When **allergies** make patients whine,
Diphenhydramine works just fine.
It blocks **histamine at H1 gates**,
And quickly calms allergic states.
Also helps with **itchy skin**,
Runny nose, and **hives** within.
In OB, it's used with care,
For **insomnia** or **nausea flare**.

It can be used to **settle sleep**,
Or help **postpartum moms** find peace.
Sometimes paired in **labor wards**,
To **relax**, or used in **nausea scores**.
Side effects are common, though:
Drowsiness is first to show.
Also **dry mouth**, **blurred vision**, too,
And **urinary retention** may come through.

It can cause **dizziness** and **fog**,
Which worsens if combined with grog.
So teach to **avoid driving** ways,
Until they know how it behaves.
There's **no Black Box Warning** on,
But still, this drug is **not a swan**
For **older adults**, or those with **fall risk**,
Due to its **anticholinergic twist**.

Contraindications may include:
Glaucoma, **BPH**, or altered mood.
And avoid in **third trimester**,
Unless provider clears the register.

Monitor **sedation**, **output**, too,
And signs of **paradoxical response** in view —
Especially in **kids**, who may go wild,
Instead of sleepy, calm, or mild.

Drug interactions are a thing,
With other meds that **drowsiness bring** —
Like **opioids**, **muscle relaxers**, **benzos** — all
Can **increase CNS depressant calls**.

DOCUSATE SODIUM (COLACE)

Stool Softener (Emollient Laxative)

When **bowels slow** and **pushing hurts**,
Docusate comes before the squirts.
It **draws in water to the stool**,
To make it soft — that's the rule.
It's **not a stimulant**, not a flush,
Just helps things pass without a rush.
Used for **postpartum moms** in pain,
Or when **opioids clog** the bowel train.

Also given **after birth**,
When **hemorrhoids** steal all joy and worth.
It helps them go without the strain,
So healing doesn't come with pain.
Side effects are pretty rare:
Maybe **cramping**, **nausea**, **gas in air**.
In high doses, **diarrhea** comes,
But most stay chill on gentle runs.

There's **no Black Box Warning** tagged,
But still make sure they're not **gagged**
From fluid loss or **GI block**,
'Cause then this med could stall the clock.
Teach to take with **fluids full**,
So it can work its hydrating pull.
And don't expect results too fast —
12 to 72 hours it lasts.

Contraindicated if you find
Bowel obstruction or **severe pain undefined**.
Don't give if they have **nausea**, too,
Without an exam to guide you through.
Monitor stool consistency,
And ask about **frequency** regularly.
It's often used on **scheduled chart**,
For patients healing every part.

DOXYCYCLINE
Tetracycline Antibiotic

When **chlamydia creeps** or **PID's rough**,
Doxycycline is strong stuff.
It blocks the bug's **protein plan**,
At the **30S ribosomal** stand.
It treats **cervicitis, acne**, too,
And **zoonotic bugs** like **tick-bite flu**.
Also used for **malaria guard**,
And **rosacea** when it hits hard.

Not for pregnancy, make it clear —
It can **stain the fetal teeth**, we fear.
Also **delays bone growth**, so pause,
Unless benefit outweighs the cause.
Side effects to teach with care:
Photosensitivity — beware!
Also **GI upset, nausea, rash**,
And rare but serious **esophagitis crash**.

Teach to take with **plenty of water**,
To keep that pill from causing slaughter.
And **don't lay down** right after the dose,
Or **throat erosion** comes real close.
No **Black Box Warning** on the chart,
But **tooth discoloration** is smart
To teach about in **kids and teens**,
And in **pregnant moms** by all means.

Contraindications include:
Pregnancy, kids under eight, that's good.
And use caution with **liver strain**,
Or **kidney issues** causing pain.
Drug interactions are a thing:
Antacids, iron, and **calcium bring**
A block to how it's **absorbed inside**,
So space them out if they collide.

DOXYLAMINE/PYRIDOXINE (DICLEGIS, BONJESTA)

When **morning sickness** won't behave,
This gentle pair can help moms brave.
Doxylamine calms the queasy tides,
While **Vitamin B6** steadies insides.
It's **FDA-approved** for NVP,
A first-line choice in pregnancy.
Safe in **early gestational days**,
When nausea hits in brutal waves.

Doxylamine is a **first-gen antihistamine**,
It blocks H1 to keep things clean.
Pyridoxine (just B6 in name),
Supports the nerves and tames the flame.
Side effects? You'll often see:
Drowsiness, dry mouth, fatigue, maybe.
Some moms feel a **bit offbeat**,
But mostly it brings gentle relief and peace.

There's **no Black Box Warning** on this pair,
But use with care and **monitor there**.
Especially with **other sedating meds**,
Like **opioids, benzos**, or **sleepy threads**.
Contraindications aren't too long:
Avoid if **MAOIs** are along.
Also take care with **severe asthma**,
Or **glaucoma** — can cause some drama.

Teach to **take it at bedtime first**,
It works best when symptoms are worst.
If **morning nausea** won't subside,
They may add a dose at the **midday tide**.
Don't crush or chew — it's delayed release,
So swallowing whole is part of the peace.
And if they feel **too sleepy** still,
Adjust the **schedule** or **dose with skill**.

DROSPIRENONE AND ETHINYL ESTRADIOL (YAZ, YASMIN)

Combined Oral Contraceptive (COC)

When birth control needs a balanced flow,
This **combo pill** is good to go.
Drospirenone and **estrogen**, too,
Help **block ovulation** right on cue.
It **suppresses LH and FSH**,
So no egg leaves its little nest.
It also **thickens cervical goo**,
So sperm can't swim their journey through.

Used for **acne, PMDD**, and **cycle pain**,
And keeping periods soft and sane.
It's **FDA-approved** for mood swings wild,
That come with cycles in many a child.
Drospirenone is **spironolactone-like**,
So it **spares potassium** — a unique spike.
It **reduces bloating, acne**, too,
But **hyperkalemia** might come through.

Side effects you'll need to note:
Nausea, headache, sore breast coat.
Breakthrough bleeding, mood shifts, yes,
And rare **clot risks**, you must assess.
Black Box Warning is on file:
Smoking + estrogen? Not in style.
Especially for **35 and older**,
That combo puts hearts in a colder folder.

Contraindications? Let's review:
→ **Clot history, liver disease**, too.
→ **Migraine with aura, renal strain**,
→ **Adrenal insufficiency**, where K+ remains.
Teach to **take it same time each day**,
Don't skip or toss your pills away.
And use **backup** if a dose is missed,
Or **vomiting** put the med at risk.

Drug interactions you should screen:
Anticonvulsants, rifampin in between.
St. John's Wort may lower effect —
So check what's herbal they might collect.

DULOXETINE (CYMBALTA)
SNRI (Serotonin-Norepinephrine Reuptake Inhibitor)

When **depression lingers**, and **pain stays tight**,
Duloxetine can help make things right.
It blocks **serotonin and norepinephrine**,
So mood and nerves feel calm again.
Used in **PPD** or **GYN pain**,
Like **fibromyalgia, pelvic strain**,
It may be used off-label too,
For **stress incontinence** breaking through.

It treats both **mood** and **muscle ache**,
Helping moms **recover** for baby's sake.
And for **anxiety**, it steadies fear,
Keeping the racing mind more clear.
Side effects are not too rare:
Nausea, dry mouth, and **sleep shifts** there.
Increased sweating, fatigue, headache,
And sometimes **appetite loss** can wake.

Black Box Warning must be known —
For **suicidal thoughts** in teens alone.
So screen for risk and **monitor close**,
Especially as doses start or dose.
Contraindications you should heed:
With **MAOIs**, you must not proceed.
Also avoid in **liver disease**,
Or **alcohol abuse** — it won't appease.

Teach to take it **same time each day**,
Don't stop abruptly — taper the way.
Relief may take **a couple weeks**,
So manage the patient's real-time peaks.
Drug interactions? Quite a few:
With **anticoagulants**, watch for bruise.
Also interacts with **NSAID meds**,
Increasing **bleeding risk** instead.

ENOXAPARIN (LOVENOX)
Low Molecular Weight Heparin (LMWH)

When **clots** are lurking out of view,
Enoxaparin pulls you through.
A **low-weight heparin**, safe and clear,
To keep **DVTs** from drawing near.
It binds to **antithrombin three**,
And blocks **factor Xa** easily.
This slows the **clotting cascade's track**,
Preventing clots from fighting back.
Used in **pregnancy** with grace,
For moms at **high-risk clotting pace**.
Also post-op or **after birth**,
To guard against **clots of worth**.
Side effects you need to spot:
Bleeding, bruising, a small **red dot**.
Injection site pain may be mild,
And **anemia** in some profiles.

Black Box Warning applies when placed
With **neuraxial blocks** (like spinals faced).
It may cause **epidural bleeds**,
So spacing doses is what OB needs.
Contraindications? Clear and true:
Active bleeding, low platelets, too.
And **hypersensitivity** to pork or meds
Like **heparin** — flag these threads.

Teach to **inject in fatty space**,
2 inches from the belly place.
Don't rub the site, let it be still —
That lowers bruising, fits the bill.
Monitor for **bleeding signs**,
Like **bloody urine**, or **darkened lines**.
No need to check **aPTT**,
But **platelets** and **CBC**? Definitely.

ERYTHROMYCIN (ERY-TAB, E.E.S., ERYTHROCIN)

Macrolide Antibiotic

Erythromycin, tried and true, A **macrolide** that fights right through. For **Gram-positives**, it's a star, And some **atypicals** from afar.
It halts the bug's **protein build**, At **50S**—that site is stilled. No synthesis, no chains begin, The **bacteria** can't grow within.
It treats **pertussis**, **strep**, and more, **Chlamydia** and **syphilis'** score. In **pregnancy**, it's often picked— When others might have risks affixed.
It's also used in **newborn's eyes**, To guard from **gonorrhea's** tries. A **prophylactic ointment** there, To keep their tiny vision clear.
But do take care with **QT time**, It may **prolong** and cause a climb. Avoid with drugs that do the same, Or **arrhythmias** may stake a claim. Common side effects you'll see: **Nausea**, **cramps**, or **diarrhea** free.
Metallic taste may spoil the bite, Or **liver enzymes** may take flight. **Hearing loss**—though rarely found, In **high doses** or if long around. And if IV's infused too fast, **Thrombophlebitis** may not pass.
Check their **liver** and **ECG**, And ask about **allergies** carefully. Don't give with **statins** in the mix— It may cause **rhabdo**, muscle tricks.
Teach to take it on **empty gut**, Unless the **GI side effects** cut. Don't crush the **enteric-coated** shell, And shake that **suspension** very well. Use caution if they're old or frail, Or if the **cardiac signs prevail**.
And **renal dosing** might be wise, If kidney **function starts to slide**. There's **no black box**, but don't relax— It's still a drug that must be tracked. With **caution**, care, and nurse's eye, We guard the dose and monitor why.
So **Erythromycin**, old but bold, Still holds its place in guidelines told. A staple of the pharmacy, With lessons still for you and me.

ESCITALOPRAM (LEXAPRO)
Selective Serotonin Reuptake Inhibitor (SSRI)

Escitalopram works with grace, To calm the mind, to slow the race. Its name is known from med school lore— The brand we call is **Lexapro**. An **SSRI**, clean and tight, It helps restore what's out of sight. By **blocking serotonin's reuptake path**, It lifts the soul from sorrow's wrath.

It's used for **MDD**, for sure, And **GAD** it may help cure. In **panic**, **OCD**, and grief, It often brings the brain relief.

Avoid if paired with **MAOIs**, Or if the **QT interval** flies. Beware of **liver damage**, too— Adjust the dose or skip it through.

Expect **nausea**, **drowsy spells**, And sometimes vivid dream-like wells. **Sexual dysfunction** may appear, And **dry mouth** makes it less than clear.

Rare but grave, **syndrome of serotonin**, Can cause the nurse to call a warnin'. **Agitation, sweat**, and **tremor rise**, With **clonus** and **a fever's cries**.

Before you start, you must assess: **EKG**, if they're at risk. Check **electrolytes—K and Mg**, To guard the heart's own harmony.

No stopping cold—don't let them try, Or **withdrawal symptoms** may apply. **Dizziness, zaps**, or mood may fall— So taper slowly, if at all.

It takes a while to show its gain, **Four to six weeks**, sometimes pain. Encourage them to wait and see, Before they quit prematurely.

Black box warning loud and clear— Watch **suicide risk**, especially near. In **teens and young adults** it spikes, So monitor for mood or psych.

Teach to avoid the **alcohol**, And tell the doc if symptoms stall. Report **worsening thoughts** right fast— Don't wait until the crisis passed.

Pregnancy? It's used with care, But **risks to baby** must be there. Weigh the needs and **watch for tone**, Especially with **SSRI alone**.

So **Lexapro**, in steady hand, Can help the hurting understand. But nurses must stay sharp and wise, To guide the path where healing lies.

ESTRADIOL
Estrogen Hormone Replacement

When **estrogen drops** and symptoms flare,
Estradiol brings balance there.
It's the **main estrogen** we make inside,
And it helps restore what's been denied.
Used for **hot flashes**, **vaginal dryness**,
Bone loss, **mood**, and **mental sharpness**.
Also part of **HRT plans**,
For **menopause**, or **gendered transitions** and scans.

It binds to **estrogen receptors** neat,
In tissues from the **brain to feet**.
Improves **lipids**, **collagen**, and **tone**,
And keeps the **vaginal walls well-grown**.
Side effects can still arise:
Nausea, breast pain, headache skies.
Mood changes, bloating, spotting, too,
And **increased clot risk** — that's your clue.

Black Box Warnings are a must:
For **stroke**, **DVT**, and **cancer trust**.
Especially when used **without progestin**,
In women with a **uterus within**.
Also flagged for **dementia risk**
When used in **older age** too brisk.
So use the **lowest dose, shortest span**,
And **review annually** the plan.
Contraindications? These apply:
Breast cancer, **clots**, or **liver's cry**.
Pregnancy, **undiagnosed bleed**,
Or **MI/stroke history** you must heed.
Teach to **rotate patches** if that's the form,
And **never place on breasts** — that's not the norm.
Or if it's **oral, take with food**,
To ease the nausea that may intrude.

Drug interactions you should know:
With **thyroid meds**, they sometimes show.
And with **CYP inducers**, the dose might fall —
So monitor levels through it all.

42

ESTRADIOL CYPIONATE / MEDROXYPROGESTERONE ACETATE (LUNELLE)

Combined Injectable Contraceptive

A **combo shot**, precise and neat, For monthly care that can't be beat. It balances two hormone tides— **Estrogen** and **progestin** sides. **Estradiol Cypionate**, smooth and slow, With **Medroxyprogesterone** in tow. Together they **suppress the egg**, And **thicken mucus**, block the leg.

Used for **contraception** once a month, An option when the pill feels blunt. It's given **IM**, a deep-set shot— Just **every 28 to 30 days on dot**.

Avoid in patients with a past Of **clots** or **stroke** that came on fast. And those with **breast cancer** or **liver disease**, Should skip this drug and find more ease.

Expect some **spotting**, maybe late, Or shifts in **weight** and **appetite**. **Headache, nausea, breast may swell**— All common, though they tend to quell.

But risks can rise in certain states: **Thromboembolism** awaits. So screen for **smoking**, age, and more— Especially over **thirty-four**. Nurses must observe with care, Ask when the **last injection** was there. Check for signs of **DVT**— Like calf pain or **swelling suddenly**.

Teach them how the cycle flows, That **protection wanes** if timing goes. A **backup method** may be wise If more than **33 days** have passed by.

This med may slightly raise the risk Of **breast cancer**, **stroke**, or **clot so brisk**. And **bone loss** comes with long-term stay— So monitor **calcium** day by day.

No STI protection, this we stress, So **condoms still** must help suppress. And if the period disappears, Rule out **pregnancy** and **calm their fears**.

There's **no black box** for Lunelle's name, But similar drugs bear **serious claim**. So nurses treat it just the same— With **vigilance**, and **informed frame**.

So when a patient wants control, But not a pill or daily role, This monthly shot, both firm and fair, Can meet her needs with nurse-led care.

ESTRADIOL TRANSDERMAL PATCH (CLIMARA, VIVELLE-DOT, MINIVELLE)

Estrogen Hormone Replacement (Transdermal)

When **hot flashes** steal the day,
The **estradiol patch** can smooth the way.
It delivers **estrogen through the skin**,
To bring hormonal balance back again.
Used for **menopause** and **HRT**,
For **trans women**, too — affirmingly.
It helps with **mood**, **sleep**, and **vaginal tone**,
And guards against **bone loss** as women age on.

It skips the **liver's first-pass round**,
So **blood clot risk** is often downed.
That makes it gentler on the whole,
For many patients, it's the goal.
Side effects to monitor:
Skin irritation, maybe sore.
Nausea, breast pain, headaches hit,
And **spotting** may occur a bit.

Black Box Warnings still apply:
Risk of **stroke**, **DVT**, and **why**
It must be used with **progestin**
If a uterus is still within.
Also flagged for **breast cancer risk**,
And **dementia** in older folks on the list.
So use the **lowest dose that works**,
And monitor for **clotting quirks**.

Contraindications include:
Pregnancy, **clots**, or **liver feud**,
Breast cancer, or **bleeding strange**,
Or a history of **MI/stroke range**.

Teach to **place the patch on clean skin**,
Not on the **breasts**, and never on thin
Broken or **irritated zones** —
Abdomen, **buttocks**, **hip**, or **flank bones**.

Change it on the **schedule right**,
Once a week or **twice** — depends on type.
Rotate sites to protect the skin,
And keep the **adhesion** firm within.

ESTRADIOL VAGINAL INSERT (VAGIFEM, IMVEXXY)

Local Estrogen Therapy (Vaginal Insert)

When **vaginal tissue** starts to thin,
And **dryness** makes it tough within,
The **estradiol insert** works just right,
To bring that tissue back to light.
It's a **low-dose local estrogen**,
That heals the walls from deep within.
Restores **moisture, pH**, and **tone**,
So postmenopausal pain is gone.

Used for **atrophy, itch**, and **burn**,
And **dyspareunia** in return.
Also helps with **urinary flare**,
Like **urgency** or **leaking there**.
It's **not for systemic hormone goals**,
Just **local action** in vaginal roles.
So it **doesn't carry full body risk**,
Like oral estrogens on the list.

Side effects are pretty rare:
Maybe **spotting, breast pain, itching** there.
Some have **headache, cramps**, or **discharge**,
But most effects are mild or marginally large.
There's **no Black Box Warning** on this form,
But general **estrogen risks** still warn.
So avoid in **cancer, DVT**,
Or **undiagnosed bleeding mystery**.

Contraindications still include:
Pregnancy, liver disease, and **clotting feud**.
Also **estrogen-sensitive cancers** stay
On the avoid list all the way.
Teach to **insert the tablet deep**,
Once a day, then **twice a week**.
Use the **applicator clean and slow**,
And let them know when results will show.

This form is **vaginal only**, true,
So teach what **symptoms** it helps undo.
And emphasize it's **not for birth**,
But for restoring tissue's worth.

45

ESTRADIOL VAGINAL RING (ESTRING, FEMRING)

Local or Systemic Estrogen Therapy (Vaginal Ring)

When **vaginal atrophy** makes life sore,
The **estradiol ring** can help restore.
It slowly releases **estrogen**,
Right where it's needed — deep within.
The **Estring** acts with **local grace**,
Just in the **vaginal tissue space**.
It eases **dryness**, **itch**, and **pain**,
And helps with **urinary urge and strain**.

The **Femring**, though, is different here —
It gives **systemic estrogen** cheer.
So it helps with **hot flashes**, too,
And more **menopausal symptoms** through.
Inserted vaginally for weeks on end,
It's **self-inserted** — no need to depend.
Usually changed **every 90 days**,
To keep those symptoms well at bay.

Side effects? They're mostly light:
Spotting, **breast tenderness**, **vaginal bite**.
Maybe **headache**, or a **ring that shifts**,
But overall, it's one that lifts.
Black Box Warning still applies,
Especially for **systemic types** (Femring guys).
Risk of **clots**, **stroke**, and **cancer scene**,
Especially when the uterus is still in between.

Contraindications you must know:
Breast cancer, clots, or **liver woe**.
Also avoid in **undiagnosed bleeds**,
Or **pregnancy** — no hormone feeds.
Teach them how to **place it clean**,
Squat or lie down, keep it routine.
No need to remove it during sex,
But if it falls out — rinse, then flex.

If **Estring**, note it's **local fare**,
So full-body risks are **mostly rare**.
If **Femring**, it's a **systemic tool**,
So **add progestin** if that's the rule.

ESTRADIOL VALERATE (DELESTROGEN)
Estrogen Hormone Replacement (Injectable)

When **estrogen** is low or gone,
Estradiol valerate moves things on.
An **injectable** form that's strong and neat,
To help bring balance back complete.
Used in **menopause** and **HRT**,
For **transgender women** affirmingly.
Also used when **periods pause**,
From **hypogonadism** or other cause.

It works like natural **estradiol**,
But in a form that **lasts** — not small.
It's given **IM** (sometimes SC),
To **mimic cycles** or dose steadily.
Side effects may still arise:
Breast tenderness, spotting, headache skies,
Mood swings, bloating, maybe **nausea**,
And rarely **thromboembolic drama**.

Black Box Warnings should be known:
For risk of **clots, stroke**, and **hormone-grown**
Endometrial cancer, especially when
Used **without progestin** now and then.
It's also flagged in **older age**,
For **dementia** and **heart disease** stage.
So use the **lowest dose that works**,
And review each year to dodge those quirks.
Contraindications to flag:
Breast cancer, clot risk, liver drag.
Also avoid with **undiagnosed bleed**,
Or in **pregnancy** — that's a need.
Teach to **rotate injection sites**,
And track for **bruising, pain**, or **fights**.
Labs may track **estradiol blood**,
To keep the levels where they should.

ETHINYL ESTRADIOL/ LEVONORGESTREL

Combined Oral Contraceptive (COC)

This classic **combo pill** is key,
For **birth control** and **hormone harmony**.
It blends **ethinyl estradiol's sway**
With **levonorgestrel** to block the way.
It **inhibits LH and FSH**,
So **ovulation** never leaves the nest.
It **thickens cervical mucus**, too,
To trap the sperm from getting through.

Used for **pregnancy prevention**, clear,
And **acne, cramps**, and **cycle gear**.
It also shows up in **Plan B**,
At **higher doses**, urgently.
Side effects you may observe:
Nausea, breast pain, spotting swerve.
Mood changes, headaches, maybe **bloat**,
And rare **clot risk** you must note.

Black Box Warning is in play —
For **smokers over 35** each day.
Risk of **stroke, DVT**, and **MI**,
Makes this warning extra high.
Contraindications must be clear:
Clots, liver disease, or **aura near**.
Breast cancer, hypertension, too —
And **undiagnosed bleeding** should stop the crew.

Teach to take it **same time daily**,
Missing pills affects it greatly.
If they **miss one**, they can recover,
But more than two? Use **backup cover**.
Drug interactions may reduce
Its power — that's important news.
Rifampin, St. John's Wort, and some **seizure meds**,
Can pull the rug from beneath its threads.

ETHINYL ESTRADIOL/ NORETHINDRONE
Combined Oral Contraceptive (COC)

When cycles stray or cramps won't ease,
This combo brings hormonal peace.
With **ethinyl estradiol** and **norethindrone**,
It helps the body find its tone.
It **inhibits LH and FSH**,
So eggs stay put inside their nest.
It also **thickens cervical goo**,
So sperm can't push their pathway through.

Used for **birth control, cycle pain, Acne, PMS,** and **period gain**.
Also part of **HRT care**,
To protect the **uterus** while estrogen's there.
Side effects you should discuss:
Nausea, bloating, tender bust.
Mood swings, headaches, spotting, too,
And rare **clot risks** that may ensue.

Black Box Warning applies again —
For **DVT, stroke,** and **cardiac strain**.
Especially when the patient's case
Involves **smoking over 35's space**.
Contraindications? Keep in view:
Breast cancer, clots, and **liver issues,** too.
Migraine with aura, pregnancy known,
Or **bleeding not yet fully shown**.
Teach to **take it at the same time** daily,
And what to do if they miss it barely.
One missed pill? **Take it quick,**
More than one? Use **backup stick**.

Drug interactions to screen:
Enzyme inducers may intervene.
Anticonvulsants, St. John's Wort,
Can make its **effectiveness fall short**.

ETHINYL ESTRADIOL/ NORGESTIMATE (ORTHO TRI-CYCLEN, SPRINTEC)

When cycles shift and breakouts bloom,
This combo helps clear up the room.
Norgestimate and **estrogen** combine,
To regulate the hormone line.
It **inhibits LH and FSH**,
So **ovulation** stays in place.
It **thickens mucus**, slows sperm's run,
And **stabilizes the endometrial fun**.

Used for **acne**, **cramps**, and **cycle care**,
And **PMS** that's hard to bear.
It's often chosen as a start,
For teens or those with acne heart.
Side effects to teach and track:
Nausea, breast pain, headache pack.
Some may spot or feel a mood,
That swings without a warning cue.

Black Box Warning applies again —

For **stroke**, **clot**, and **cardiac strain**.
Especially if they **smoke and age**,
Past **35** — that turns the page.
Contraindications you must list:
Breast cancer, clots, or liver cyst.
Uncontrolled BP, **pregnancy near**,
Or **migraine aura** — avoid it here.

Teach to **take it daily, same time**,
And **what to do** if they miss the line.
One missed pill? Take it soon.
More than one? **Back it with a spoon**
(aka backup method in tune ☺).
Drug interactions may occur:
Like **rifampin**, or **St. John's herb**.
Anticonvulsants can drop its power,
So double-check the med list hour by hour.

ETONOGESTREL IMPLANT (NEXPLANON)

Progestin-Only Long-Acting Reversible Contraceptive (LARC)

A tiny rod with major might,
Etonogestrel stops sperm in flight.
It goes **inside the upper arm**,
And guards from pregnancy with charm.
It **inhibits ovulation** first,
And **thickens mucus** at the cervix burst.
The **endometrium thins**, too — that's key,
So there's no place for eggs to be.

Used for **contraception long**,
It lasts **three years** and stays strong.
Safe in **breastfeeding, teen**, or **new**,
And **fertility returns** when it's removed, too.
Side effects you need to track:
Irregular bleeding may come back.
Some get **acne, mood shifts**, or **weight**,
Or **ovarian cysts** at a mild rate.

There's **no Black Box Warning** on the tag,
But like all progestins, screen and flag.
Teach they might not **bleed each month**,
But that's expected — not a stunt.
Contraindications you should know:
Active clots, liver tumors, or **cancer's show**.
And if they've had **allergy** before,
To the implant or the materials core.
Placed with care in a **sterile field**,
The inner arm is where it's sealed.
Local anesthesia, quick and done —
And **palpate the rod** once it's begun.
Teach to avoid **heavy lift or strain**,
For **24 hours**, keep it plain.
And if **they can't feel it** down the line,
They should call the doc to realign.

FAMCICLOVIR (FAMVIR)
Antiviral (Purine Nucleoside Analog)

When **herpes flares** or **shingles sting**,
Famciclovir can calm the thing.
It's an **antiviral** in disguise,
Converted in the **liver** to fight and rise.
It becomes **penciclovir**, fast and strong,
To stop the **virus** from growing long.
It blocks **viral DNA replication**,
Halts infection's full foundation.

Used for **herpes zoster**, **HSV**,
Cold sores, genital lesions, you'll see.
Also used in **pregnancy**,
For **suppressive therapy** safely.
Side effects you might find:
Headache, nausea, tired mind.
GI upset, dizziness,
And rare **rash** or **allergic mess**.

There's **no Black Box Warning** stamped,
But still, be careful where it's camped.
It's best to start at **first outbreak**,
For faster healing's give and take.
Contraindications? Few are known,
Except if **hypersensitivity** is shown.
Use caution in **renal decline**,
And adjust the dose to keep it fine.

Teach to take it **with or without food**,
And stick to timing — that's the mood.
It's **not a cure**, just holds things back,
And lowers risk of **outbreak attack**.
Also teach about **safe sex**, too,
Even without lesions in view.
And if for **suppression late in term**,
It may protect the newborn worm.

FLUCONAZOLE (DIFLUCAN)
Azole Antifungal

When **yeast takes hold** and won't let go,
Fluconazole delivers the blow.
It blocks **ergosterol production**,
Which halts the fungal cell's construction.
Used for **vaginal yeast** with flair,
Just **one dose** often gets it there.
Also treats **thrush, fungal spread**,
And infections that go systemic instead.

Side effects may still appear:
Nausea, headache, GI cheer.
Liver enzymes may go high,
So monitor **AST/ALT** nearby.
There's **no Black Box Warning** on this med,
But watch for risks in **liver** spread.
And in **pregnancy**, it gets complex —
Single-dose OK, but **high-dose vex**.

Avoid **chronic use** in pregnant care,
Unless the benefit is truly rare.
High doses may cause **birth defects**,
So follow **guidelines** — no regrets.
Contraindications you must know:
Allergy to azoles is a no-go.
And use with caution in **QT-prolonged**,
Or **arrhythmias** that could go wrong.

Teach to **avoid alcohol swigs**,
It may enhance the **liver digs**.
And space it out from **CYP3A4 meds**,
Like **warfarin, seizure drugs**, or **statin threads**.
It's **oral or IV**, both well-tolerated,
But for **yeast infections**, it's often celebrated.
Remind them that **relief takes time** —
One or two days before they shine.

FLUCONAZOLE VAGINAL TABLET

When **yeast infections** make things rough,
And creams alone aren't strong enough,
The **vaginal tablet** hits the zone —
Right at the source, not system-wide grown.
It works like oral **fluconazole**,
But used **vaginally** to meet the goal.
It blocks **ergosterol** in the wall,
So fungal cells can't grow at all.

It's used for **vaginal candidiasis**,
To ease the **itch**, the **burn**, the **swollenness**.
Inserted deep just **once at night**,
It brings relief without the bite.
Side effects are mostly mild:
Local irritation, discharge styled.
Some may feel a **pelvic cramp**,
Or **itching** near the placement camp.

There's **no Black Box Warning** here,
But standard **azole cautions** appear.
Avoid in **pregnancy high-dose**,
Unless the provider gives the close.
Contraindications are rare to see —
Just **allergy to azoles** is key.
And those with **recurrent yeast flares**,
Should follow up to rule out scares.
Teach to insert it **deep inside**,
Before bed is best — then rest and ride.

Don't use **tampons** while it's in,
And **abstain from sex** 'til healing begins.
It's **not the same** as oral form,
Though both treat yeast — different norms.
This route stays **local, low absorption**,
Less risk of systemic contortions.

FLUOXETINE (PROZAC)
SSRI (Selective Serotonin Reuptake Inhibitor)

When **mood drops low** and tears don't stop,
Fluoxetine can help things pop.
It **blocks serotonin reuptake tight**,
To lift the mind and bring back light.
Used for **depression, PMDD, Anxiety,** and **OCD**.
In **postpartum care**, it plays a role,
To help new moms regain control.

Side effects may come and go:
Insomnia, headache, GI flow.
Dry mouth, sweating, sexual decline,
And **nervousness** in some design.
Black Box Warning stands tall:
For **suicidal thoughts** — especially small.
In **teens and young adults**, beware —
Monitor mood shifts with patient care.

Contraindications include:
Recent **MAOIs** — that's no good.
It needs a **14-day washout clear**,
To avoid **serotonin syndrome fear**.
Teach that relief may take **weeks to show**,
4 to 6 weeks before it flows.
Don't stop abruptly or skip a beat —
Withdrawal symptoms aren't so sweet.

It has a **long half-life**, true —
So it may stay **longer in you**.
That makes it good for **missed pill days**,
But not ideal if switching ways.
Drug interactions to be aware:
With **NSAIDs, anticoags** — bleeding flare.
And watch when taken with **other serotonins**,
To avoid **serotonin storm** within.

FOLIC ACID (VITAMIN B9)

When **babies grow** and **cells divide**,
Folic acid works inside.
It builds up **DNA and nerves**,
And gives the fetus what it deserves.
It's used in **pregnancy** with pride,
To stop **neural tube defects** from inside.
Like **spina bifida, anencephaly**,
This vitamin helps prevent them early.

Also treats **megaloblastic strain**,
A type of **anemia** moms may gain.
It helps with **RBCs** being made,
So energy doesn't start to fade.
Side effects are rare and small:
Just **GI upset** — not much at all.
It's well-tolerated in every phase,
From preconception through birth days.

There's **no Black Box Warning** here,
But use with care and guidelines clear.
Too much may **mask B12 decline**,
So check both levels if not fine.
Contraindications? None are strong,
Unless **hypersensitivity** tags along.
It's safe in **pregnancy and lactation**,
And part of every **prenatal foundation**.

Teach to take it **every day**,
Even before conception's way.
The usual dose is **400 mcg**,
But high-risk folks may need a tug:
4 mg daily if risks are high —
Like **previous NTDs**, or **anticonvulsants** nearby.
And **dietary folate** helps it land,
In **leafy greens, beans**, and grains on hand.

GABAPENTIN (NEURONTIN)
Anticonvulsant / Neuropathic Pain Agent

When **nerves misfire** or **pain won't fade**,
Gabapentin comes to aid.
It calms the **nervous system's spark**,
And brings relief when nights get dark.
It mimics **GABA** in some ways,
Though not a direct GABA blaze.
It blocks **calcium channels** tight,
To soothe **nerve pain** both day and night.

Used in **chronic pelvic pain**,
Or **neuropathy** that won't wane.
It's also used when **hot flashes** hit,
Especially when **HRT won't fit**.
Side effects that may appear:
Drowsiness, dizziness, thinking unclear.
Fatigue, weight gain, and **swelling legs**,
May cause a shift in comfort pegs.

There's **no Black Box Warning** here,
But still, some things must be clear:
Watch for **mood or behavior change**,
And rare **suicidal thoughts** in range.
Contraindications? Not too many,
But caution in **renal impairment** plenty.
Adjust the dose if kidneys lag,
To avoid a toxic drag.

Teach to take it **every night**,
And not to stop it in a fright.
Taper slowly, don't go cold —
Withdrawal risks must be controlled.
It may enhance **CNS depressants**,
So avoid **alcohol** or **benzo presence**.
Teach patients not to **drive too quick**,
Until they know if it makes them sick.

GONADOTROPINS (E.G., FSH, LH, HCG)
Ovulation Induction Agents / Reproductive Hormones

Gonadotropins, a powerful trio, To help the **egg and follicle grow**. They mimic what the body makes— And give **fertility** its stakes.
There's **FSH** to start the race, It **stimulates the follicle's space**. Then **LH** surges to the sky, To **trigger ovulation's high**.
And **hCG** steps in to stand For **LH's** job with steady hand. It tells the **ovary**, "Now, release"— And helps the **luteal phase** find peace.
These hormones help in **ART**, Like **IVF** or when cycles start. They're used when natural cues are low, To make the **eggs mature and grow**.
But nurses must beware the risk— Of **OHSS**, that swelling twist. When ovaries **over-respond**, It's more than just a hopeful bond.
Bloating, pain, and **weight that jumps**, **Shortness of breath** or fluid clumps. This syndrome needs a cautious eye— In rare cases, it can terrify.
Side effects include **mood shifts**, **Multiple births**, and **pelvic tiffs**. Also watch for **injection site pain**, And **hormone storms** that wax and wane.
Assess the **baseline hormone set**, And **ultrasound** to catch each threat. Watch **estradiol**—don't let it soar, That's how **OHSS** knocks at the door.
Teach patients how it's all timed tight— **FSH first**, then **trigger at night**. Ovulation comes in **a day or so**, So they must follow protocol. Explain the signs that must be told— **Chest pain, swelling, fever, cold**. Stress **hydration**, gentle care, And call the doc if things impair.
No **black box**, but don't assume— These meds can bring both joy and gloom. It's **hope in vials**, well understood, With **nurse-led safety** making good.
So **Gonadotropins** pave the way, For families hoping every day. But with their power, side by side, Comes **nursing skill** as trusted guide.

HYDRALAZINE (APRESOLINE)
Direct Vasodilator / Antihypertensive

Hydralazine, a name to know, When **blood pressure** starts to overflow. It works right on the **arteries**, wide, To let the **pressure drop** and slide.
Its brand is known as **Apresoline**, A med to keep those numbers clean. It causes **vasodilation fast**, By **relaxing smooth muscle** to the last.
It's used for **hypertension's** spike, Or **preeclampsia** when things aren't right. In **pregnancy**, it's often picked— A **safe choice** when the pressure's kicked.
It may be used in **heart failure**, too, When afterload needs lowered through. In **crisis**, it may be IV— To drop that pressure urgently.
Watch out for **headache**, pounding loud, Or **palpitations** in a crowd. **Tachycardia** may appear, As the **heart reacts** to dropping gear.
Side effects can also show As **nausea, sweats,** or **flush and glow**. Some feel **dizzy, weak**, or pale— So rise up slow, and grab the rail.
A rare but serious thing to find: **Lupus-like syndrome** in due time. **Butterfly rash, joint pain, fever**— Symptoms that might linger, ever.
Monitor that **BP close**, Before you give the ordered dose. Check **HR**, too—don't miss the trend— Watch for **reflex tachycardia's bend**.
Taper slow—don't stop too quick, Or **rebound hypertension** might stick. Educate to **take as told**, And store the meds away from cold.

Tell patients not to drive too fast Until the **drowsy fog** has passed. And if their **ankles swell or ache**, They should call for **fluid's sake**.
No **black box warning**, but still wise— To treat this drug with watchful eyes. Especially when **IV's pushed**, Stay ready if the BP's rushed.
Hydralazine, a gentle push, To bring down pressure's harmful crush. With nurse at side, dose by dose, It guards the heart and keeps it close.

HEPARIN
Anticoagulant (Indirect Thrombin Inhibitor)

When **clots** are forming deep inside,
Heparin helps to turn the tide.
It binds to **antithrombin III**
And blocks **factor Xa** and **IIa** (thrombin) free.
It's used in **pregnancy** with care,
Because it doesn't **cross the placenta** there.
Great for moms at **clotting risk**,
Like **history of DVT**, or **lupus twist**.

Also used for **prophylaxis** post-op,
To keep the clotting risks to a drop.
And in **IV form**, it works fast,
But **subcutaneously**, it also lasts.
Side effects to watch and know:
Bleeding, bruising, platelet low.
Rarely causes **HIT** to rise —
That's **heparin-induced thrombocytopenia** in disguise.

Black Box Warning is in place
For **epidurals and spinal space** —
It may cause **bleeding near the cord**,
So time the dose with strict accord.
Contraindications? Yes, indeed:
Active bleeding, or **platelets freed**.
Also avoid with **HIT on record**,
Or **hypersensitivity** noted or stored.

Monitor labs for safety signs:
aPTT for IV lines.
Not needed for the **subQ way**,
But still check **platelets** every day.
Teach to rotate **injection spots**,
Avoid **NSAIDs**, and **bleeding clots**.
And if they're **going home with Lovenox**,
Be sure they know it's **not the same box**.

HYDROCODONE/ ACETAMINOPHEN (NORCO, VICODIN, LORTAB)

Opioid Analgesic + Non-Opioid Analgesic Combo

When **postpartum pain** is sharp and deep,
This combo helps new moms find sleep.
Hydrocodone blocks the pain so loud,
While **acetaminophen** joins the crowd.
It binds to **mu receptors** tight,
To **alter how the brain feels fright**.
The **acetaminophen** works on the side,
To lower the **fever** and pain that's wide.

Used for **C-section, episiotomy**,
Or **after surgery recovery**.
Short-term use is what we say,
To **manage pain the safer way**.
Side effects are common, though:
Drowsiness, dizziness, GI slow.
Constipation, nausea, dry mouth, itch,
And **sedation** can flip the switch.

Black Box Warning is clear and bold:
Risk of **respiratory depression** told.
Also flagged for **addiction's grip**,
And **liver damage** if **Tylenol tips**.
Contraindications? Yes, we know:
Severe respiratory issues in tow.
And caution if they're **opioid naïve**,
Or with other meds that **CNS deceive**.

Teach them not to **double dose**,
Especially when **Tylenol's close**.
Avoid **alcohol**, and watch their state —
No driving if they're feeling sedate.
Monitor pain and **respiratory rate**,
Bowel movements, and how they relate.
And taper down when **pain is mild**,
To keep the risk low for mom and child.

HYDROXYZINE (VISTARIL, ATARAX)

First-Generation Antihistamine / Anxiolytic

When **itching strikes** or **nerves run high**,
Hydroxyzine is worth a try.
It's an **antihistamine** at its core,
But it **calms the brain** and **settles the roar**.
Used for **anxiety, nausea**, too,
Allergies, hives, or a **pre-op view**.
It's also helpful **before birth**,
To **sedate** and show what calm is worth.

It blocks **H1 receptors**, slows the tide,
With **anticholinergic drift inside**.
So it helps with **sleep, itch**, and **chill**,
When **benzos** aren't the right-fit pill.
Side effects to keep in mind:
Drowsiness, dry mouth, foggy kind.
Constipation, dizzy, blurred sight,
And **urine retention** may take flight.

There's **no Black Box Warning** known,
But teach with care when it's shown.
Don't mix with **alcohol, opioids, benzos**,
Or anything that **slows the CNS flow**.
Contraindications you must flag:
First trimester pregnancy bag
(Vistaril is often avoided then),
Prolonged QT, or **elder risk**,
Or **hypersensitivity**, not on your list.

Teach it's given **oral or IM deep**,
(But **never IV** — safety to keep!)
Help them rest when tension's tall,
Or when **itchy skin** drives up the wall.

IBUPROFEN

When **pain** and **inflammation** rise,
Ibuprofen is your prize.
It blocks **COX enzymes**, lowers the flame,
And **prostaglandins** lose their game.
It's used for **cramps**, **C-section pain**,
Afterbirth aches, or **fever strain**.
Also great for **headache days**,
And **swelling** in a dozen ways.

Side effects may come in time:
GI upset, **ulcers**, **bleeding line**.
Heartburn, **nausea**, and **dizzy light**,
And rare **renal issues** out of sight.
Black Box Warning is stamped in place:
Risk of **MI** and **stroke** to face.
Especially with **long-term use**,
And in those with a **cardiac caboose**.

Also flagged for **GI bleeds**,
Ulcers, **perforation** — serious needs.
So teach to **take it with some food**,
To guard the stomach and boost the mood.
Contraindications? Take note:
GI ulcers, or if they've wrote
A history of **kidney disease**,
Or **NSAID allergy** — avoid with ease.

In **pregnancy**, caution appears:
Avoid in **third trimester years**.
It may close the **ductus arteriosus** gate,
And cause **bleeding** at a higher rate.
Teach to **limit alcohol**, too,
To protect the **stomach lining** through.
And don't stack it with **other NSAIDs** near —
It won't boost pain, just risk severe.

INDOMETHACIN (INDOCIN)
NSAID (Nonsteroidal Anti-Inflammatory Drug)

When **labor starts a bit too quick**,
Indomethacin can do the trick.
It blocks **prostaglandins** with might,
To keep the uterus calm and tight.
Used as a **tocolytic tool**,
Before **32 weeks** — that's the rule.
Also treats **period pain** with skill,
And **inflammation** that won't stay still.

Side effects? You should know:
Nausea, drowsiness, GI blow.
Heartburn, headache, dizzy sway,
And sometimes **bleeding** comes your way.
Black Box Warning flags the risk
Of **GI bleeds, stroke**, or **cardiac twist**.
Especially with **chronic use**,
So limit length — don't let it loose.

In **pregnancy**, it's **used with care**,
But not beyond **week 32's stare**.
It can cause **ductus arteriosus close**,
And **oligohydramnios** — that's no joke.
Contraindications? Yes, they stay:
Peptic ulcer, GI bleed, asthma play.
Kidney disease, or **NSAID flair**,
Or if they've had a **stroke affair**.

Teach to take it **with some food**,
To help the GI tract stay in a good mood.
And monitor for **urine drop**,
In case the kidneys start to flop.
It's often used **short-term and fast**,
To help contractions **not to last**.
Then stopped before those risks grow wide —
Just long enough to turn the tide.

INSULIN
Hormone / Antidiabetic Agent

When **blood sugar** rises past the line,
Insulin helps it realign.
It moves **glucose into the cells**,
Where energy and balance dwells.
Used in **pregnancy** with pride,
When diet and exercise can't guide.
It's the gold standard in **GDM**,
To protect both **baby** and **the stem**.

Also used in **type 1, type 2**,
And in **L&D** if sugars flew.
Given **subQ** or sometimes **IV**,
It works fast or gradually.
There are **basal, bolus, short**, and **long**,
Each one playing a different song.
Like **regular, NPH**, or **glargine's call**,
Each one helps prevent the fall.

Side effects to watch and note:
Hypoglycemia gets the vote.
Sweating, shaky, blurred out talk,
And **confusion** on a dizzy walk.
Weight gain, lipodystrophy too,
If they don't **rotate sites** like they should do.
Allergic reactions are very rare,
But monitor still — and always care.

There's **no Black Box Warning** here,
But safety still is crystal clear:
Check **BG levels** night and day,
To keep those spikes and crashes away.

Contraindications? Not really so,
Unless they're allergic — then it's a no.
But be cautious with **renal decline**,
As **insulin clearance** may realign.

Teach to **store it right, draw it clean**,
And follow their **sliding scale routine**.
Help them spot those **lows and highs**,
And keep some **glucose** nearby.

IRON SUPPLEMENTS (FERROUS SULFATE, FERROUS GLUCONATE, ETC.)

Mineral / Hematinic

When **fatigue** hits hard and **labs look pale**,
Iron supplements help tip the scale.
They build up **hemoglobin's might**,
To carry **oxygen** day and night.
Used in **pregnancy** when demand is high,
To help the **RBCs multiply**.
Also key for **postpartum moms**,
Whose **blood loss** may ring silent alarms.

They help treat **iron-deficiency**,
From **diet**, **bleeding**, or **delivery**.
And boost reserves to help restore
The strength that moms are longing for.
Side effects are common here:
Constipation, **dark stools**, and **GI smear**.
Some feel **nausea**, **cramps**, or **bloating**,
And **metallic taste** that feels demoting.

There's **no Black Box Warning** stamped,
But overuse can **iron-clamp**.
So store away from **children's hand**,
To avoid a **toxic iron land**.
Contraindications are few and mild:
Avoid in **hemochromatosis wild**,
Or if there's **iron overload disease**,
Or **anemias not from iron's needs**.

Teach to **take it on an empty gut**,
But with **vitamin C** to help it strut.
Avoid antacids, **dairy**, **coffee**, too —
They block the **absorption** coming through.
Teach about **black stools** — that's okay,
And **fiber** helps keep cramps at bay.
Let them know it works real slow,
It takes **weeks to months** for levels to grow.

LABETALOL (TRANDATE)
Beta Blocker (Nonselective + Alpha-1 Blocker)

When **BP climbs** and won't come down,
Labetalol helps calm the crown.
It blocks both **beta** and **alpha-1**,
So **pressure drops**, but heart's not done.
Used in **pregnancy** with care,
To treat **chronic hypertension** there.
Also used when **preeclampsia** spikes,
Or **severe-range pressures** sound the mics.

It lowers **HR** and **vascular tone**,
But **keeps the uterus safe alone**.
That's why it's used in OB lands —
It doesn't slow the **placenta's plans**.
Side effects may show in view:
Fatigue, dizzy, GI flu.
Bradycardia, cold hands or feet,
And **orthostatic drops** that aren't sweet.

Black Box Warning applies if stopped
Abruptly — the BP might pop.
So taper slow when therapy ends,
To avoid rebound BP trends.
Contraindications include:
Asthma, bradycardia, and that mood
Where **heart block** or **shock** is near —
Don't give if output disappears.

Teach to check their **pulse and rate**,
Before each dose — don't medicate

If the **HR's low** or **pressure's dropped**,
Call the provider — the dose gets stopped.
It can be given **PO** or **IV push**,
For urgent needs or steady hush.
And in **labor**, it plays a role,
To keep **BP** under control.

LAMOTRIGINE (LAMICTAL)
Anticonvulsant / Mood Stabilizer

When **seizures spark** or **moods swing low**,
Lamotrigine helps steady the flow.
It blocks **sodium channels** in the brain,
And quiets that **electric train**.
Used in **epilepsy** with grace,
And in **bipolar disorder's case**.
It's often chosen in **pregnancy**,
For **mood and seizure stability**.

Side effects you must discuss:
Dizziness, blurred vision, GI fuss.
Headache, tiredness, sleepy drag,
And a rare but serious **skin rash flag**.
Black Box Warning is clear and loud:
For **Stevens-Johnson Syndrome** in the crowd.
So titrate slow and watch the skin —
Any rash should be reported in.

Contraindications are quite few,
But allergies to the med won't do.
Use caution in **renal** or **hepatic strain**,
And monitor **levels** if they complain.
Teach to take it **every day**,
Same time — no skipping on the way.
Abrupt withdrawal could bring a storm,
So taper down to keep them warm.

It's often used with **other meds**,
So watch for **interactions** in their threads.

Estrogen can **lower lamotrigine**,
So **dose adjustments** may step in.
In **pregnancy**, it's sometimes best,
With **fewer defects** than the rest.
But always weigh the **risk vs. goal**,
And check levels as a routine role.

LETROZOLE (FEMARA)
Aromatase Inhibitor

When **ovulation's** gone off track,
Letrozole helps to bring it back.
It blocks **aromatase** — the key,
So **estrogen drops** temporarily.
That drop tells **FSH to rise**,
To grow a follicle of prize.
Used in **PCOS** and more,
To open up the **fertile door**.

Taken just for **five short days**,
In early cycle **timed phase**.
Often **days 3 through 7** or **5 to 9**,
Then wait for **ovulation's sign**.
Side effects can still be felt:
Hot flashes, **headache**, **sweating melt**.
Dizziness, **fatigue**, and **bloating**, too,
And rare **ovarian cysts** may come through.

There's **no Black Box Warning** placed,
But still, **use caution** just in case.
It's not for use in those already **pregnant**,
So check **before** the pills are sent.
Contraindications you should know:
Premenopausal cancer without clear go.
Or **known hypersensitivity**,
Or **liver dysfunction** in the history.

Teach they may feel **emotional tide**,
As hormones swing and levels slide.
Multiple follicles may grow,
So **twins or more** may start to show.
It's also used in **cancer care**,
For **estrogen-driven tumors** there.
But in fertility, it's short and sweet —
A quiet boost to help **ovulation repeat**.

LEUPROLIDE (LUPRON)

When **estrogen drives the pain too far**,
Leuprolide steps in like a star.
It mimics **GnRH** at first,
Then **shuts down hormones** to quench the burst.
It's used for **fibroids**, **endometriosis**,
And **precocious puberty diagnosis**.
It's also part of **IVF prep**,
To time the cycle with careful step.

At first it causes **hormone flare**,
Then **suppression** kicks in fair and square.
So **LH and FSH** fall low,
And **estrogen/progesterone** cease to flow.
Side effects you must explain:
Hot flashes, mood swings, vaginal strain.
Bone loss, too, with use that's long,
So **add-back therapy** may belong.

No Black Box Warning, but take care —
Osteoporosis risk hangs in the air.
So **calcium + vitamin D** should be,
Part of the treatment plan you see.
Contraindications? A few to name:
Pregnancy, or **vaginal bleeding** with no name.
Breastfeeding, or **allergy past**,
Or **severe bone loss** that's been cast.

Teach about the **menopause-like** feel,
And how the **periods may stop** or peel.
It may be **IM or subcut** injected,
With **monthly or depot** forms selected.
Used **short-term** for GYN pain,
Until **surgery** or longer plans explain.
And for **IVF**, it helps control
The timing for that embryo goal.

LEVONORGESTREL
Progestin (Synthetic Progesterone)

When **pregnancy's not in the plan today**,
Levonorgestrel clears the way.
It mimics **progesterone's control**,
And keeps the **uterus on a steady role**.
It **inhibits ovulation** when it's timed,
And **thickens mucus** every time.
It thins the **endometrial bed**,
So there's no soft place for an egg to tread.

Used in many forms you'll see:
→ **Progestin-only pills** (POP) for daily.
→ **IUDs** like **Mirena**, **Kyleena**, **Skyla**,
→ Or **Plan B** — emergency style-a.
In **IUDs**, it slowly releases near,
To last **3 to 8 years** — safe and clear.
In **Plan B**, it's used high-dose,
To stop ovulation before it goes.

Side effects? Here's what's known:
Irregular bleeding, **cramps**, **moan**.
Breast tenderness, **acne**, **mood**,
Sometimes **weight gain** joins the brood.
There's **no Black Box Warning** on its face,
But still use caution in each case.
For **ectopic pregnancy**, teach signs,
Like **unilateral pain** and **fainting lines**.

Contraindications to note:
Pregnancy known, or **liver bloat**,
Breast cancer, or a **uterine fibroid**
That **distorts the cavity** — avoid deployed.
Teach how the **timing** really counts,
Especially when using **Plan B amounts**.
It works best in the **first 72**,
But may help up to **day five**, too.

And if they use the **IUD style**,
Remind it might change **bleeding awhile**.
Periods may **lighten** or even stop —
That's expected with this hormone drop.

LEVOTHYROXINE (SYNTHROID, LEVOXYL, EUTHYROX)

Thyroid Hormone (T4 Replacement)

When the **thyroid slows** and **energy drops**,
Levothyroxine fills the gaps and stops.
It mimics **T4** the body makes,
To boost the **metabolism stakes**.
Used for **primary hypothyroid**,
From **Hashimoto's** or **gland destroyed**.
Also used in **pregnancy**,
To keep **mom and baby's brain** on beat.

Side effects from too much dose:
Tachycardia, **heat**, and **nervous host**.
Weight loss, sweating, restless nights,
Like you're running marathons in tights.
There's **no Black Box Warning**, true,
But dosing must be **watched right through**.
Start low, go slow — it's wise to say,
Especially in those with **heart display**.

Contraindications you must screen:
Acute MI, or **adrenal not seen**.
And if the patient has **hyperthyroid**,
They don't need more — that plan's void.
Teach to take it **on an empty gut**,
In the **morning**, same time in the rut.
Wait **30 to 60 minutes** to eat,
Or absorption won't be complete.
Avoid with **calcium**, **iron**, or **soy**,
They block the dose — not a joy.
Space those out by **4 hours long**,
To keep the medication strong.
Monitor TSH to guide the plan,
Adjust the dose as symptoms span.
In **pregnancy**, they'll need more fast,
Thyroid demand can quickly blast.

LIDOCAINE (XYLOCAINE)
Local Anesthetic / Antiarrhythmic (Class 1B)

When **numbness** is the goal on hand,
Lidocaine is in demand.
It **blocks sodium channels fast**,
So nerve signals simply don't get past.
Used in **labor** and **OB repairs**,
Like **episiotomies** or **tears**.
Also used for **IV lines**,
Or numbing skin for **little signs**.

It may be used **topical or injected**,
And must be **dosed and well-selected**.
Too much can cause a toxic turn,
So **safety checks** are your concern.
Side effects? They're rare, but real:
Tingling, tremors, or a strange feel.
At high doses: **seizures, slurred speech**,
Bradycardia, or a **CNS breach**.

In **IV form**, it also plays
A role in **cardiac arrest phase** —
It's a **Class 1B antiarrhythmic**,
Used when **ventricles go ballistic**.
There's **no Black Box Warning** marked,
But **toxicity** can still be sparked.
Especially when given **too much, too fast**,
So **aspirate before** you let it blast.

Contraindications? A few to name:
Allergy to amides, or **heart block game**.
Caution with **liver disease**,
Since metabolism may freeze.

Teach it may **burn or sting at first**,
But then the numbness starts to burst.
If they feel **ringing in the ear**,
Or feel **confused**, call help near.

LORATADINE (CLARITIN)

When **pollen flies** or **hives appear**,
Loratadine brings breathing clear.
It blocks the **H1 histamine spot**,
To cool the sneeze and itching blot.
Used for **allergic rhinitis** mild,
Or **urticaria** when skin runs wild.
And safe for **pregnancy** to boot —
For stuffy nose or itchy suit.

It's a **non-drowsy antihistamine**,
Unlike **diphenhydramine's dream**.
So moms can take it through the day,
And still keep fatigue at bay.
Side effects are pretty tame:
Headache, dry mouth, tired frame.
But no sedation for most who try —
That's why it's often the first to fly.

There's **no Black Box Warning** here,
But don't exceed the dose, be clear.
It's **once daily, 10 mg** is norm,
Unless the provider shifts the form.
Contraindications are rare,
Just **allergy to it** — so take care.
Use caution in **hepatic strain**,
And adjust if liver enzymes wane.

Teach they can take it **with or without food**,
And it won't mess with the sleepy mood.
Great for **seasonal sneezes**,
wheals, and **rash**,
Without the sedation crash.

MAGNESIUM SULFATE
Electrolyte / Anticonvulsant / Tocolytic

When **preeclampsia's pressure climbs**,
Magnesium sulfate buys some time.
It **relaxes nerves and muscle tone**,
To keep **seizures down** and **tension shown**.
It's used for **eclampsia** to prevent,
And **preterm labor** when contractions are sent.
Also used for **brain protection**,
If birth comes early — **neural connection**.

It **blocks neuromuscular twitch**,
By **calcium channel ditch**.
This slows the body's firing rate,
And helps prevent a seizing fate.
Side effects? Be sure to teach:
Flushing, nausea, lethargy reach.
Respiratory depression is the fear —
So monitor closely while it's near.

There's **no Black Box Warning**, but —
Toxicity is a serious rut.
Watch for **loss of deep reflex signs**,
And **respiratory rate below 12 lines**.
Contraindications to know:
Heart block, renal failure, or **low RR flow**.
And if **calcium levels dip too low**,
This drug could make the symptoms grow.

Antidote? Keep it close in hand —
Calcium gluconate as planned.
Give **IV slowly**, don't delay,
If toxicity comes into play.
Teach the patient what to feel:
Warmth, muscle weakness, heavy heel.
And let them know that while it's slow,
It helps keep **seizures** from the show.

MEDROXYPROGESTERONE ACETATE (DEPO-PROVERA)

Progestin / Hormone Replacement / Injectable Contraceptive

When **estrogen's not the way to go**,
Depo-Provera steals the show.
A **progestin-only shot** that stays,
To block **ovulation** for **90 days**.
It **inhibits LH and FSH**,
And **thickens mucus** at the cervix edge.
It thins the lining, stops the egg,
And **suppresses periods** without a peg.

Used for **birth control** that's long,
Amenorrhea for those who long
To stop their cycles, **bleed less**, rest,
Or treat **endometriosis distress**.
Side effects you must discuss:
Weight gain, mood swings, acne fuss.
Headache, hair loss, delayed return
Of fertility — a patient concern.

Black Box Warning stands in place:
Long-term use may **thin bone space**.
So limit to **2 years** when you're able,
Unless no other options are on the table.
Contraindications you'll screen:
Breast cancer, or **liver disease** seen.
Also avoid if there's a **clotting past**,
Or **undiagnosed bleeding** that could last.

Teach to **get the shot every 3 months**,
And don't delay or take the chance.
They may have **irregular bleeds** at first,
But later periods may disperse.
It's given **deep IM** in the **glute**,
Or **subcutaneously**, both routes suit.
Counsel about **calcium, vitamin D**,
To protect the bones long-term and free.

MEDROXYPROGESTERONE (ORAL - PROVERA)

Progestin / Hormone Replacement Therapy (HRT)

When **cycles stop** or **bleeding pours**,
Provera comes and steadies the doors.
It mimics **progesterone's** effect,
To **shed the lining**, clear and correct.
Used for **amenorrhea, AUB**,
To bring a **period** back gently.
Also paired with **estrogen's might**,
To **protect the uterus** day and night.

In **HRT**, it's a key support,
To keep the **endometrium** from cancer's court.
Given in **short bursts** or **cyclic style**,
To regulate cycles and calm the mile.
Side effects to teach with care:
Bloating, mood swings, acne flare.
Breast tenderness, headaches, too,
And maybe some **mid-cycle goo**.

There's **no Black Box Warning** on its own,
But when used with **estrogen tone**,
Black Box risks come into play —
Clots, strokes, and **breast cancer** sway.
Contraindications you must review:
Pregnancy, liver disease, or **clot history**, too.
Undiagnosed bleeding? Investigate.
Breast cancer past? Avoid this fate.

Teach to take it **same time each day**,
Usually for **5 to 14 days** in a play.
And if the **period doesn't start**,
Let the provider check the chart.
It may cause **withdrawal bleed**,
So prepare them for what that may lead.
And in **PCOS**, it's often the key,
To cycle hormones and regulate free.

MEFENAMIC ACID (PONSTEL)

NSAID (Nonsteroidal Anti-Inflammatory Drug)

When **period pain** comes sharp and loud,
Mefenamic acid stands out proud.
It blocks the **COX enzymes** with might,
To calm the cramps and ease the fight.
Used for **dysmenorrhea**, clear,
And **heavy bleeding** once a year.
Also treats **mild pain** and strain,
When inflammation fans the flame.

Side effects you might expect:
Nausea, headache, GI defect.
Heartburn, dizziness, and **gas**,
Or **diarrhea** that may not pass.
Black Box Warning is in play,
For **cardiac** and **GI risks** that stay.
MI, stroke, and **bleeding gut**,
Especially if used in chronic rut.

Contraindications? You must know:
Ulcers, GI bleeds, or **renal blow**.
Late pregnancy is also flagged,
Since it may close the **ductus sagged**.
Teach to take it **with some food**,
To help the stomach handle the mood.
And don't mix with **other NSAIDs** near,
That raises risk — be extra clear.

Often taken **at period start**,
To soothe the **cramping uterus heart**.
Not for long-term use or daily —
Just **short bursts** when cramps hit gaily.

METFORMIN (GLUCOPHAGE)
Biguanide / Antidiabetic Agent

When **insulin's high** and cells resist,
Metformin helps to clear the mist.
It lowers **glucose made by the liver**,
And helps the **muscles** act as giver.
Used in **type 2 diabetes care**,
And **GDM** when diet's unfair.
It's also used in **PCOS**,
To help with **cycles**, **weight**, and stress.

Improves **ovulation** in some plans,
So **fertility** gets helping hands.
It may be used in **IVF prep**,
Or to get periods back in step.
Side effects you should expect:
GI upset, **metallic speck**.
Nausea, diarrhea, bloating show,
Especially when doses start out low.

There's **no Black Box Warning** here,
But watch for **lactic acidosis fear**.
Rare but serious, so take care,
With **renal disease** or **oxygen despair**.
Contraindications? Let's be wise:
Kidney disease, or if **creatinine's high**.
Alcohol abuse, or **sepsis on** —
Those are cases where it's gone.

Teach to take it **with a meal**,
To help the stomach better deal.
And don't take right before or after
IV contrast — wait to capture.
It doesn't cause **hypoglycemia** solo,
But may if used with **insulin's flow**.
Monitor **glucose**, track the signs,
And reassess at A1C times.

METHYLDOPA (ALDOMET)
Alpha-2 Adrenergic Agonist

When **blood pressure climbs** and baby's near,
Methyldopa is calm and clear.
It works in the **brain** to turn things low,
So **sympathetic tone** won't grow.
It stimulates **alpha-2**,
To stop the nerves from breaking through.
This lowers **BP** slow and mild,
Making it safe for **mom and child**.

Used for **chronic HTN in preg**,
It won't impair the **placenta leg**.
It's not as fast as **labetalol**,
But works long-term to **guard them all**.
Side effects? There may be:
Fatigue, drowsiness, dry mouth spree.
Depression, bradycardia,
And **fluid retention** now and ah.

There's **no Black Box Warning** tagged,
But still, this med can leave folks dragged.
So check on mood and mental tone,
Especially if they feel alone.
Contraindications to screen:
Liver disease, or **MAOI scene**.
Also watch in **depression's case**,
It may return and slow their pace.

Teach to take it **twice per day**,
And not to skip or walk away.
Warn about the **sedating feel**,
Especially behind the wheel.
Monitor **BP trends, labs**, and signs,
AST/ALT, from time to time.
And if the BP's not controlled,
Consider adding meds more bold.

METHYLERGONOVINE (METHERGINE)

Ergot Alkaloid / Uterotonic Agent

When **bleeding flows** and won't slow down,
Methylergonovine turns it around.
It clamps the **uterus firm and tight**,
To stop that **postpartum bleeding fight**.
It works on **smooth muscle tone**,
To make the **uterine fundus like stone**.
Used in **PPH** when **atony hits**,
This drug can stop those hemorrhage fits.

Given **IM**, or sometimes **PO**,
Or **IV in emergencies**, slow.
Onset's fast, and action is strong —
But use it right — don't get it wrong.
Side effects you'll need to share:
Hypertension, nausea, cramping flare.
Headache, dizziness, and **chest pain**,
From too much squeeze in the vessel lane.

Black Box Warning? Nope — not quite,
But serious risks are still in sight.
Don't give with **hypertension, pre-eclampsia**,
Or **heart disease** — that's the idea.
Contraindications to know:
Chronic HTN, CAD in tow,
Stroke history, or **hepatic strain**,
Could worsen with this uterine gain.

Teach it's used **after delivery's done**,
To keep the **uterus firm as one**.
They may feel **cramping** — that's okay,
It means the **bleeding's held at bay**.
Monitor **bleeding, fundus height**,
And **BP** closely every night.
It's not for labor — not its lane,
It's postpartum when we call its name.

METOCLOPRAMIDE (REGLAN)

Prokinetic / Antiemetic / Dopamine Antagonist

When **nausea lingers** and food won't move,
Metoclopramide gets in the groove.
It blocks **dopamine** in the gut and brain,
So **nausea**, **vomit**, and **bloat** wane.
Used in **pregnancy** with care,
When **morning sickness** fills the air.
Also treats **GERD** and **delayed empty**,
When food feels stuck and **stomach's hefty**.

Sometimes used to **boost breast milk**,
By raising **prolactin**, smooth as silk.
Though not first-line, it may be tried
When **lactation's lagging** far and wide.
Side effects that may be seen:
Fatigue, **restlessness**, or a twitchy lean.
Diarrhea, **sedation**, and more rare —
Tardive dyskinesia — beware.

Black Box Warning rings aloud:
Tardive dyskinesia can be proud.
A **permanent twitch** from long-term use —
So short-term only, not abuse.
Contraindications you must scan:
Seizures, **GI bleed**, or **Parkinson's plan**.
Also avoid with **bowel obstruction**,
Or **pheochromocytoma** function.

Teach to take it **before they eat**,
Usually **30 minutes** — that's neat.
Let them know it may cause **drowsy heads**,
So caution with driving or sleepy meds.
Monitor for **extrapyramidal signs**,
Like **tremors**, **stiffness**, **spasming lines**.
And if symptoms worsen fast,
Stop the drug — don't let it last.

METRONIDAZOLE (FLAGYL)
Nitroimidazole Antibiotic / Antiprotozoal

When **vaginal discharge** turns off track,
Metronidazole brings balance back.
It fights **anaerobes** and **protozoa**,
Like **BV** and **trich** — you'll thank the flora.
It's first-line for **bacterial vaginosis**,
And **trichomoniasis** with a bonus.
Also used in **PID fights**,
And **GI bugs** like **C. diff** bites.

It disrupts **DNA inside**,
So microbes can't grow, no matter how they tried.
It's available **oral**, **IV**, or **vaginal gel**,
So treatment can match the symptoms well.
Side effects you might expect:
Metallic taste, GI defect.
Nausea, cramps, or **darkened pee**,
And **dizziness** occasionally.

No Black Box Warning per the chart,
But a **key teaching point** stands out from the start:
No alcohol during use, it's true —
Or **disulfiram reaction** may come through.
Flushing, vomiting, pounding head,
Like you're allergic to wine instead.
So teach to wait **48 hours post-last dose**,
Before drinking anything close.

Contraindications to hold:
First-trimester trich, if not told.
Use caution in **liver disease**,
And with **blood dyscrasias** if you please.
Teach to finish the **full med course**,
Even if symptoms lose their force.
And partner treatment is a must —
For **trich**, treat both or break the trust.

MICONAZOLE (MONISTAT)
Azole Antifungal (Imidazole Class)

When **itching burns** and **yeast runs wild**,
Miconazole brings comfort mild.
It stops the fungus at the source,
So healing takes a gentle course.
It blocks **ergosterol's creation**,
Disrupts the **fungal cell foundation**.
Used in **vaginal candidiasis**,
To fight that common **yeast distress**.

Available **OTC** in creams or tabs,
Or **suppositories** for nighttime grabs.
Often used in **1, 3, or 7-day** sets,
Depending on how strong the infection gets.
Side effects are mainly local:
Burning, **itching**, **vaginal focal**.
Some may feel a little **sting**,
But overall, relief it brings.

There's **no Black Box Warning** on the page,
And it's **safe in pregnancy** at the right stage.
In **pregnancy**, the **7-day form** is best —
It's gentle, thorough, and passes the test.
Contraindications are few and light:
Just avoid if **allergic** — that's your right.
Teach not to use with **tampons near**,
Or **vaginal sex** 'til meds are clear.
Tell them to insert it **deep at night**,
And wear a **liner** if discharge takes flight.
Relief comes fast, but still complete
The full course so yeast can't repeat.

MISOPROSTOL (CYTOTEC)
Prostaglandin E1 Analog / Uterotonic Agent

When the **uterus needs a gentle nudge**,
Misoprostol gives it a budge.
It **ripens cervix**, **contracts the womb**,
And helps the body make more room.
Used for **induction** when labor stalls,
Or **miscarriage care** when no one calls.
Also treats **postpartum bleeds**,
When the uterus won't meet tone needs.

It mimics **prostaglandin flair**,
To **soften the cervix** and **make muscles care**.
It can be given **buccal**, **rectal**, **vaginal**, **oral**,
Its routes are flexible, never quarrel.
Side effects you might see:
Cramping, **nausea**, **chills**, **fever spree**.
Diarrhea, **shivering**, and **GI pain**,
But most effects are short and plain.

There's **no Black Box Warning**, but still —
This med requires **watchful skill**.
Too much can cause **uterine tachysystole**,
Or **rupture risk** if scar's in the role.
Contraindications to assess:
Previous C-section? Use with finesse.
Hypersensitivity, or **labor too fast**,
Can make this drug a risky cast.

Monitor contractions and baby's tone,
And **reassess if hypertones** are shown.
In **PPH**, it's given **rectally** post,
When **oxytocin** alone can't boast.
Teach that **cramping** will be real,
That's the med helping things heal.
And when used for **loss or abortion's plan**,
Offer **supportive care** — a compassionate hand.

85

NAPROXEN (ALEVE, NAPROSYN)

NSAID (Nonsteroidal Anti-Inflammatory Drug)

When **cramps** hit hard and bring the ache,
Naproxen helps the muscles break.
It blocks **COX enzymes** head-to-head,
To stop the **prostaglandins' spread**.
Used in **dysmenorrhea** strong,
And **endometriosis pain** that's long.
Also for **postpartum aches** or swell,
When pain relief is needed well.

It reduces **inflammation** fast,
And helps the relief **longer last**.
More potent than **ibuprofen** for some,
But still needs care with how it's done.
Side effects you need to teach:
GI upset, nausea, ulcers reach.
Dizziness, headache, fluid hold,
And **increased BP** as it unfolds.

Black Box Warning is on file:
For **GI bleeds**, and **cardiac style**.
Risk of **stroke** and **MI** may grow,
So use the **lowest dose** you know.
Contraindications to keep clear:
Ulcers, GI bleeds, or **NSAID fear**.
Renal disease, third-trimester date,
May close the **ductus** — not so great.

Teach to take it **with a meal**,
To protect the stomach from the deal.
And don't mix with **other NSAIDs**, too —
That combo isn't good for you.
Often given on a **schedule timed**,
For **menstrual pain**, it's right in line.
It helps reduce the **flow and sting**,
And lets the uterus do its thing.

NIFEDIPINE (PROCARDIA)
Calcium Channel Blocker (CCB)

When **contractions start** before they should,
Nifedipine can do some good.
It blocks **calcium from muscle walls**,
So **uterine tone** and **pressure falls**.
Used to treat **preterm labor flow**,
To help the pregnancy **longer go**.
Also used in **chronic HTN**,
Or **preeclampsia** now and then.

It relaxes **vascular smooth muscle**,
And **uterine cramps**, so moms don't hustle.
PO route is how it's given,
Short-acting tabs, not time-driven.
Side effects you might observe:
Headache, flushing, nausea swerve.
Hypotension, dizzy, and **palpitation**,
May come with vessel relaxation.

There's **no Black Box Warning** tied,
But **BP drops** can override.
So watch for **orthostatic dips**,
And **tachycardia** as it slips.
Contraindications to screen:
Hypotension, or if **shock is seen**.
Heart failure, MI, or **aortic flow**,
All need a different med to go.

Teach to rise up **slow from bed**,
And monitor what **side effects** are said.
No **grapefruit juice**, and space with care
From other **BP meds** they bear.
In **labor**, check for **uterine tone**,
And **fetal heart** before it's shown.
It's a **tocolytic** that buys some time,
To get those **steroids in on time**.

NITROFURANTOIN
(MACROBID, MACRODANTIN)
Urinary Tract Antibiotic

When **urinary burning** won't let go,
Nitrofurantoin runs the show.
It fights infection **in the bladder**,
Without disturbing systems that matter.
Used for **UTIs**, both big and small,
And safe in **pregnancy** for most all.
Also used when **bacteria hide**,
But **symptoms haven't yet arrived**.

It damages **bacterial DNA**,
So bugs can't grow or find their way.
It's **urine-specific**, targeted fine —
So it's **not for pyelo** or kidney line.
Side effects are mostly tame:
Nausea, headache, brown urine game.
Flatulence, dizziness, sometimes **rash**,
But reactions are mild and tend to pass.

No **Black Box Warning**, but wait —
Use caution near **term or neonate**.
At **38 weeks or beyond**, it's true,
There's **hemolytic risk** if baby's due.
Contraindications you should note:
CrCl below 30 — nope, no boat.
Also avoid in **first trimester**
If there's a **safer option** to enter.

Teach to take it **with a meal**,
To help the GI tract feel more chill.
And **complete the full course** even when

Symptoms stop — or it might come again.
It's often dosed as **Macrobid**,
Twice a day, for just a bid.
Don't use for **pyelonephritis pain**,
It won't reach kidneys — not its lane.

NORETHINDRONE
Progestin-Only Contraceptive / Hormone Therapy

When **estrogen's not a safe bet**,
Norethindrone is your best yet.
A **progestin-only** daily pill,
To **regulate cycles** or **bleeding still**.
Used for **birth control** with grace,
And in **perimenopause** to brace.
Also helps in **endometriosis**,
By calming uterine overgrowth's focus.

It **inhibits ovulation** (but not always),
So **mucus thickens** and **cycles phase**.
It keeps the **endometrium thin**,
So spotting stops and cycles win.
Side effects you might explain:
Irregular bleeding, weighty gain,
Headache, bloating, mood shift, too,
And sometimes **acne** coming through.

There's **no Black Box Warning** solo,
But when used with **estrogen's flow**,
⚠ Risks for **clots** and **stroke** can rise —
So it's safer on its own in some eyes.
Contraindications include:
Pregnancy, or **liver feud**,
Undiagnosed bleeding, or **breast CA**,
Or **clots** that have not gone away.

Teach to take it **same time daily**,
Within 3 hours — not so gaily.
Missing it can **drop control**,
So strict routine is part of the role.

Great for **breastfeeding** moms who need
A **safe and hormone-light** birth control lead.
And in those with **migraine aura signs**,
It's preferred over estrogen lines.

NORETHISTERONE ENANTATE (NET-EN)
Progestin-Only Injectable Contraceptive

Norethisterone Enantate, bold, A **progestin shot** that nurses hold. It stops **ovulation** in its track, And thickens **cervical mucus's back**. Known as **Net-En**, it's injected deep, A **long-acting dose** that doesn't sleep. It's given every **two months** straight— To keep **unplanned pregnancies** off the plate.
It's used where **access** may be tough, A method **simple, strong, and rough**. For those who need a **quiet plan**, Without a pill or daily scan.
It's **contraindicated** in the case Of **liver disease**, or **cancer's trace**. And don't combine with **clotting past**— As **VTE risk** may rise fast. Expect **spotting**, maybe late, A **missed period** or altered state. **Weight gain**, **headache**, or **breast sore**, And mood swings may knock at the door.
But rare effects may still arise— Like **vision change** or **jaundiced eyes**. So check for **aura**, **sudden pain**, Or **depression** that won't explain. Nurses must assess with care— **Pregnancy ruled out**, med prepared. **Deep IM** into the glute, Not for the arm, nor something cute. Teach to come **on time, not late**, Or **backup birth control** is fate. If more than **14 days** go past, A **pregnancy test** is ordered fast. No protection from **STI**, So teach the **condom's role** and why. And if the **bleeding** is too strong, They should report—it could be wrong.

No **black box warning** for this med, But counsel what the research said— Long-term use may **lower bones**, So watch for **fractures**, aches, and groans.
And when they want to **try conceiving**, It may take months before retrieving The natural rhythm, back again— Be patient with the body's trend.
So **Net-En** stands where pills may fail, A quiet shot to guide the trail. But with its strength, comes nurse's role— To guard the cycle and the goal.

ONDANSETRON (ZOFRAN)
Antiemetic / 5-HT3 Serotonin Receptor Antagonist

When **morning sickness** won't let go,
Ondansetron helps the nausea slow.
It blocks the brain's **serotonin beat**,
To calm the gut and bring relief sweet.
Used in **pregnancy** to treat
Nausea that knocks moms off their feet.
Also used when **post-op** feels grim,
Or **chemo** makes the stomach spin.

It works at the **CTZ brain zone**,
And on the **vagus nerve** alone.
To stop that queasy, swirling track,
And bring the appetite safely back.
Side effects? They're mild and rare:
Headache, **fatigue**, and **constipation flair**.
Occasionally, a **QT prolong**,
So **EKG** if they're at risk long.

There's **no Black Box Warning** in place,
But still, assess the **rhythm space**.
In **pregnancy**, some debate remains —
Use when needed, weigh the gains.
Contraindications? A few to check:
Congenital long QT on deck.
Or **hypersensitivity** from prior use,
Or **electrolyte imbalances** on the loose.

Teach to take it **before they eat**,
Or when that queasy wave repeats.
Often **oral**, **IV**, or **ODT**,
To fit whatever route they need it to be.

ORMELOXIFENE (CENTCHROMAN / SAHELI)

Selective Estrogen Receptor Modulator (SERM)

When **hormonal options** don't align,
Ormeloxifene steps in just fine.
A **weekly pill** to block conception,
Without full hormonal intervention.
It **blocks estrogen** in breast and womb,
But lets it work in bone to bloom.
So periods lighten, flow gets tame,
And **fibroid symptoms** lose their flame.

Used for **DUB** or **cycle distress**,
Or as a **non-hormonal contraceptiveness**.
No daily pills or mood swing fright —
Just **twice a week**, then **once**, done right.
Side effects are usually rare:
Some get **delayed periods** or mild flare.
Occasional **headache, bloating,** slight,
But most report they're feeling right.

There's **no Black Box Warning** at this time,
But research's scope is still mid-climb.
And while it's safe in **most who try**,
It's **not used during pregnancy's sky**.
Contraindications to screen:
Pregnancy, lactation, clotting scene,
Liver disease, or if the goal
Is **quick conception** — not its role.

Teach to take it **twice a week** for 3,
Then **once a week** is all they need.
Start on **day one of the bleed**,
And back it up until it leads.

OXYCODONE/ ACETAMINOPHEN (PERCOCET)

Opioid Analgesic + Non-Opioid Analgesic Combo

When **postpartum pain** runs deep and wide,
Percocet helps to turn the tide.
Oxycodone stops pain at the brain,
While **acetaminophen** cools the flame.
Used for **C-section, laceration,**
Or **post-op OB situations.**
It tackles pain too strong for just Tylenol,
But still requires **careful call.**

It binds to **mu receptors** tight,
To **block pain signals** day and night.
The **acetaminophen** adds the spark
To make relief both quick and sharp.
Side effects to keep in view:
Drowsiness, dizziness, itching, too.
Constipation, nausea, respiratory slow,
And rare reactions that may grow.

Black Box Warning is in place:
For **addiction, abuse,** and **fatal pace.**
Also for **respiratory depression,**
And **liver damage** from acetaminophen.
Contraindications you must screen:
Severe respiratory issues in between.
Avoid with **liver disease** or **opioid allergy,**
And monitor with care in any **analgesic synergy.**

Teach to **avoid alcohol** at all,
And take it on the **lowest call.**
Caution if driving or caring for babe,
As **sedation** may crash the wave.
Monitor **pain, RR,** and signs of misuse,
And **bowel movements** — don't let them lose.
Use short-term only, then taper slow,
To keep dependence from gaining a go.

OXYTOCIN (PITOCIN)
Uterotonic / Hormone

When **labor's stalled** or needs a start,
Oxytocin plays a key part.
It mimics what the **body makes**,
To help the uterus **contract in waves**.
It binds to **oxytocin sites**,
To trigger **contractions** strong and tight.
Used for **induction, augmentation**, too —
And **PPH** when bleeding's due.

It's given **IV**, in **careful titration**,
With **fetal monitoring** and close observation.
It's never pushed — that would be wrong —
It's dripped in slow and built up strong.
Side effects may come in tow:
Uterine tachysystole.
Water intoxication if run long,
From its **antidiuretic song**.

No Black Box Warning, but still —
It's **high alert**, so use with skill.
Too much can lead to **uterine rupture**,
Or **fetal distress** that interrupts her.
Contraindications you must know:
CPD, malpresentation show,
Fetal distress before the drip,
Or if a **classical scar** may rip.

Monitor **contraction patterns** close,
And stop the line if they **overdose**.
Watch **fetal heart rate, resting tone**,
And **vitals** — never leave her alone.
It's also used **after birth's done**,
To help the **uterus stay firm as one**.
It clamps down vessels, stops the flow —
A **PPH rescue** you'll want to know.

PAROXETINE (PAXIL)
SSRI (Selective Serotonin Reuptake Inhibitor)

When **mood is low** and thoughts won't lift,
Paroxetine can give a shift.
It blocks **serotonin's reuptake track**,
To help bring **balance and calmness back**.
Used for **depression, panic, grief**,
And **PMDD** to bring relief.
It's also used postpartum when
Anxiety or sadness won't end.

Side effects may come at start:
Nausea, dry mouth, heavy heart.
Drowsiness, sweating, weight gain, too,
And **sexual dysfunction** out of the blue.
Black Box Warning on display:
Suicidal thoughts in youth may sway.
So monitor mood with care and grace,
Especially in the early phase.

⊘ In **pregnancy**, use with care —
Category D, so be aware.
Linked to **heart defects**, especially first,
So often **avoided** unless symptoms are worse.
Contraindications? Let's be wise:
No **MAOIs** — a risk that's high.
A **14-day washout** must be done,
Or **serotonin syndrome** may come.

Teach that **effects may take 4 weeks**,
And don't stop suddenly when relief peaks.
Taper slowly, don't withdraw,
To avoid that emotional seesaw.

PENICILLIN V (PEN-VEE K)
Beta-Lactam Antibiotic (Natural Penicillin)

When **gram-positive bugs** invade the scene,
Penicillin V helps keep things clean.
It breaks the **bacterial cell wall lines**,
So germs can't grow or hold their signs.
Used for **strep throat**, **mild skin sores**,
And **dental abscess** behind closed doors.
Also safe for **pregnancy care**,
For simple infections that linger there.

It's an **oral form**, not IV,
So mild to moderate bugs it frees.
Not for **severe** or **systemic spread**,
But great for **strep** or **gum pain dread**.
Side effects? Keep this in mind:
Nausea, **diarrhea**, **rash** you'll find.
Yeast infections may appear,
So warn about the flora here.

There's **no Black Box Warning** on the chart,
But **allergic reactions** are a serious part.
Anaphylaxis, though rare, is real —
So screen their **allergy history deal**.
Contraindications to track:
Penicillin allergy — don't look back.
Use caution in those with **renal strain**,
And space with meals to reduce pain.

Teach to take it **all the way**,
Even if symptoms go away.
Skipping doses or stopping quick
Might let the bugs come back thick.

PRAMOXINE
Topical Local Anesthetic

When **itching, burning,** or **sting won't stop**,
Pramoxine gives the symptoms a drop.
It numbs the skin with a gentle block,
To calm the nerves and soothe the shock.
Used in **hemorrhoids** and **perineal pain**,
After **delivery, tears,** or **strain**.
Also helps with **vaginal itch**,
Without the need for steroid switch.

It **blocks sodium channels** fast,
So nerve signals can't be passed.
Applied in **creams, wipes,** or **gels**,
It's found in many OTC shells.
Side effects are rarely loud:
Redness, burning, or **rash allowed**.
But reactions are usually mild and brief,
Just monitor for **relief or grief**.

There's **no Black Box Warning** in its lane,
But always watch for **skin reaction pain**.
And avoid use on **broken skin**,
Where absorption risks could begin.
Contraindications are few and light:
Just avoid if there's **allergy** in sight.
And don't apply too wide or deep,
Or systemic side effects might creep.

Teach to use it **as directed**,
And **wash hands** when it's ejected.
It's safe for **pregnancy, post-birth, too,**
When itching makes them feel unglued.

PROGESTERONE (PROMETRIUM)

Progestin / Hormone Replacement

When the **uterus preps for life inside**,
Progesterone helps turn the tide.
It **builds the lining**, keeps it thick,
And makes implantation really stick.
It's used to **regulate the flow**,
Or help when **periods come and go**.
Also used for **IVF support**,
And **preventing loss** of pregnancy's start.

In those with **short cervix** showing risk,
It helps the uterus **stay tight and brisk**.
And in **HRT**, it's used to shield
The uterus when **estrogen is revealed**.
Routes include **vaginal, oral, IM**,
It all depends on the patient's plan.
From **gels and suppositories** to **oily shots**,
Each form supports the uterine plots.

Side effects are hormone-esque:
Bloating, tender breasts, and **restless rest**.
Mood swings, spotting, nausea, too —
And **sleepiness** that can ensue.
There's **no Black Box Warning** alone,
But in **combination**, risk is shown.
When paired with **estrogen**, risk can rise
For **clots, stroke**, and **cancer** ties.

Contraindications include:
Undiagnosed bleeding, or **liver feud**.
Avoid in **breast cancer, clots**, or **stroke**,
Unless cleared under specialist scope.
Teach to use it **just as planned**,
And know it's part of **pregnancy's stand**.
If they feel **dizzy, sad**, or **weak**,
Let the provider take a peek.

PROMETHAZINE (PHENERGAN)

Antiemetic / Antihistamine (First-Generation H1 Blocker)

When **nausea strikes** and won't back down,
Promethazine helps calm the frown.
It blocks **histamine in the brain**,
To settle **vomit**, **itch**, or **strain**.
Used in **pregnancy** to ease the day,
When **morning sickness** gets in the way.
Also helps with **motion dread**,
Or **allergies** from toes to head.

It works in the **CTZ brain zone**,
And **vestibular nerves** that moan and groan.
Given **oral, rectal, IV,** or **IM**,
It's flexible depending on the gem.
Side effects? Oh yes, a few:
Sedation, dry mouth, dizzy, too.
Blurred vision, hypotension dips,
And **extrapyramidal** (though rare) blips.

Black Box Warning for kids exists:
In those under **2**, it must be missed.
Risk of **severe respiratory depression**,
So avoid in that age without question.
Contraindications to keep in sight:
Coma, CNS depression — not right.
And use with care in **asthma's crew**,
It may worsen the airway, too.

Teach to avoid **driving or stairs**,
Until they know how it impairs.
It's **stronger** than options like Zofran's grace,
But **drowsiness** may slow the pace.

PSYLLIUM (METAMUCIL)
Bulk-Forming Laxative / Fiber Supplement

When **pregnancy slows the bowel parade**,
Psyllium helps the path be laid.
It's **fiber-rich** and **plant-based, too**,
To bulk the stool and help it move through.
It draws in **water**, makes stool **soft**,
And helps it glide with just a cough.
Used for **hemorrhoids**, **postpartum strain**,
And when **iron supplements clog the train**.

It's safe for **daily use in preg**,
With fluids high and feet with peg.
Great for **routine bowel flow**,
Without the cramping harsher meds show.
Side effects are mild and light:
Gas, bloating, or a **fullness fight**.
If taken without water—beware!
Choking risk is lurking there.

There's **no Black Box Warning** tied,
But water must be **amplified**.
8 ounces with each dose or so,
To help the fibers **safely grow**.
Contraindications? Only few:
GI obstruction, or if they **can't chew**.
If they've had **trouble swallowing down**,
Choose a different fiber crown.

Teach to mix it **well and quick**,
Then drink it down — don't let it stick.
And give it time — it's not instant magic,
But works best when **hydration's not tragic**.

RALOXIFENE (EVISTA)
SERM (Selective Estrogen Receptor Modulator)

When **bones grow thin** and **estrogen's gone**,
Raloxifene helps keep them strong.
It mimics **estrogen** in **bone and heart**,
But blocks it where **cancer could start**.
It's used in **postmenopausal years**,
To **strengthen bones** and **calm the fears**
Of **vertebral fracture** or **breast CA**,
When hormone therapy's not okay.

It **stimulates estrogen** in bone,
To slow **resorption** that's overgrown.
But blocks it in the **uterine line**,
So endometrial risk stays fine.
Side effects to educate:
Hot flashes, leg cramps, weighty gait.
Risk of **clot (DVT/PE)** is real,
So assess for **mobility and heel**.

Black Box Warning is loud and clear:
Clots and **stroke** can still appear.
Especially in those with risk before,
Like **immobility, surgery**, or more.
Contraindications? Yes indeed:
Pregnancy, clotting history, liver need.
And don't use in **childbearing frame** —
It's strictly for **postmenopause** name.

Teach to **walk and move** each day,
To lower clot risks along the way.
And **take it daily, food or not**,
With calcium and D to keep bones hot.

RHO(D) IMMUNE GLOBULIN (RHOGAM)

Immune Globulin / Anti-Rh Antibody

When **mom is Rh-negative** but baby's not,
RhoGAM steps in to guard the spot.
It stops her body from making the fight
Against **Rh-positive red cells** in sight.
It **binds fetal Rh+ cells** real fast,
Before mom's immune response can last.
So she won't make **antibodies** strong,
That could harm a baby later on.

Given at 28 weeks routinely,
And again **within 72 hours** cleanly,
After birth if baby's **Rh+ crew**,
To keep mom's future **pregnancies safe too.**
Also given when there's **mix of blood**,
Like:
- **Amniocentesis**
- **Trauma thud**
- **Abortion, ectopic**, or **bleed**,
- That's all when RhoGAM may be the need.

Side effects are mild and rare:
Injection site pain, fever flare.
Very rarely an **allergic spike**,
But most tolerate it quite alike.
There's **no Black Box Warning** on this med,
But monitor if **reactions** are said.
And always **type and screen** before,
To ensure **mom's Rh status** is sure.

Contraindications to know:
Rh-positive moms, or if **antibodies show.**
If she's already **sensitized**,
It's too late — the risk has crystallized.
Teach this drug is **not for harm**,
It's meant to keep **future babies calm.**
And it's **not a blood product risk**,
It's screened and cleaned, no need to frisk.

SERTRALINE (ZOLOFT)
SSRI (Selective Serotonin Reuptake Inhibitor)

When **mood drops low** and tears don't rest,
Sertraline helps moms feel their best.
It blocks the brain's **serotonin slide**,
So balance can be realigned inside.
Used for **PMDD**, **depression**, too,
Postpartum sadness, and **anxious view**.
Also great for **panic**, **grief**,
To help them breathe and find relief.

Side effects you may review:
Nausea, **sweating**, **tremors**, too.
Sexual dysfunction, **GI play**,
And **headaches** that may go away.
Black Box Warning is there:
For **suicidal thoughts**, so show care.
Especially in **young adults**,
Monitor mood and verbal jolts.

Pregnancy-safe? Among the best —

Often **first-line** when moms feel stressed.
No strong ties to **major harm**,
Though **newborn jitter** can raise alarm.
Contraindications? They are slim:
Avoid with **MAOIs** on a whim.
Use caution with **liver strain**,
And always **taper off** the train.

Teach that **relief may take some time** —

About **4 to 6 weeks** feels sublime.
Don't stop cold — withdrawal's rough,
So always **wean** when it's enough.

SIMETHICONE (GAS-X, MYLICON)
Antiflatulent / Anti-Gas Agent

When **bloating builds** and bellies ache,
Simethicone gives bubbles a break.
It **breaks surface tension** down in the gut,
So gas can move — no painful rut.
Used for **pregnancy** when food feels stuck,
Or after **C-sections** to ease the muck.
Also safe for **newborn tummies**,
When trapped air makes cranky mommies.

It works by **breaking up gas bubbles**,
To ease the stretch and gut-like troubles.
It doesn't **prevent** or **block new air**,
It just helps **relieve what's already there**.
Side effects are rare and light,
It's usually tolerated just right.
Maybe **mild nausea** or a shift,
But no sedation, no big rift.

There's **no Black Box Warning** at all,
And it's safe in doses **big or small**.
No known **drug interactions** bother,
And it's gentle enough for **newborns and mothers**.
Contraindications? Nearly none.
Unless allergic — then don't run.
No systemic absorption's true —
It acts right where digestion blew.
Teach to take it **after meals**,
Or **at bedtime** if discomfort steals.
It comes in **chewables**, **drops**, or **gel**,
So pick the form that suits them well.

SULFAMETHOXAZOLE/ TRIMETHOPRIM (BACTRIM, SEPTRA)

Sulfonamide + Folic Acid Antagonist (Antibiotic Combo)

When **bacteria spread** and won't behave,
SMX/TMP comes in to save.
It blocks **folic acid** from being made,
So germs can't grow or invade.
Used for **UTIs**, **MRSA**, **bronchitis**, too,
And **acne, ear**, or **bowel bug flu**.
Also used for **PCP prevention**,
In those with low immune retention.

Sulfamethoxazole stops the chain,
While **Trimethoprim** blocks the same.
Together they hit the bug in sync —
A **double blockade** in a blink.
Side effects to keep in sight:
Rash, GI upset, light sensitivity light.
Crystalluria — so push fluids through,
And **bone marrow suppression** (though rare) is true.

No Black Box Warning, but know:
There's risk for **Stevens-Johnson show**.
And in **late pregnancy**, risks are real —
Kernicterus can make it a bad deal.
Contraindications to screen with care:
Pregnancy (esp. third trimester) beware.
Also avoid in **folate deficiency**,
G6PD deficiency, or **kidney injury**.
Teach to drink **lots of water** clear,
To stop the crystals from forming near.
Take it **with food** if GI pain,
And **avoid sun** to stop the burn stain.

TAMOXIFEN (NOLVADEX)
SERM (Selective Estrogen Receptor Modulator)

When **estrogen feeds the cancer's flame**,
Tamoxifen steps into the game.
It **blocks receptors** in breast cells tight,
To **slow the growth** and win the fight.
Used for **ER+ breast cancer care**,
To **treat** or **prevent** it in those who dare.
Also used in **fertility lanes**,
To help with **ovulation gains**.

In **the uterus** and **bone**, it plays
Estrogen's role in helpful ways.
But in the **breast**, it firmly stops
That hormone's growth-supporting hops.
Side effects to warn with grace:
Hot flashes, **mood swings**, **swelling face**.
Nausea, **vaginal discharge**, too,
And **period changes** coming through.

Black Box Warning is real and bold:
Risk of **uterine cancer**, **clots**, and **stroke** told.
So monitor for **leg pain**, **chest**, or **bleeds**,
And report unusual **pelvic needs**.
Contraindications you should know:
Pregnancy is a solid no.
Also avoid in **clotting disease**,
Or **history of DVTs**.

Teach to take it **same time daily**,
And know that **treatment plans** may vary.
Usually **5 years** for cancer care,
Though some may go **10 years there**.
And if it's used to **boost a cycle**,
Ovulation may spike like a rifle.
But warn that **twins or more** may show —
As hormone levels start to grow.

TERBUTALINE (BRETHINE)
Beta-2 Adrenergic Agonist / Tocolytic

When **contractions start too soon to show**,
Terbutaline says **"not yet — no go."**
It binds to **beta-2** so smooth,
To help the uterus **rest and soothe**.
Used in **preterm labor's early storm**,
To delay delivery and keep things warm.
It buys time for **steroids to kick**,
So baby's lungs develop quick.

It relaxes **smooth muscle**, not just womb,
But **lungs and heart** can feel the boom.
That's why side effects may appear,
So monitor closely — stay near.
Side effects? They can be strong:
Tachycardia, tremor, palpitations along.
Nervousness, hypotension, chest pain,
And **hyperglycemia** may explain.

Black Box Warning — take note:
Oral and injectable long-term use gets a vote
Against routine use for stopping birth —
Due to **heart risks** and **maternal dearth**.
Contraindications to keep clear:
Cardiac disease, HTN, or **diabetes gear.**
Also avoid with **tachycardic signs**,
Or in **bleeding, infection,** or **unripe times.**

Teach it's given **subcutaneously**,
Or sometimes **IV in emergencies**.
Monitor **HR, BP,** and tone,
And listen if **mom says something's wrong**.
Watch for **fetal tachycardia**, too —
And stop the med if symptoms brew.
It's not for use all long-term day,
Just **short bursts** to push birth delay.

TERCONAZOLE (TERAZOL)

Azole Antifungal

When **yeast takes hold** and causes strife,
Terconazole brings back normal life.
It stops the fungus **from growing more**,
By damaging its **cell wall core**.
It's used for **vaginal candidiasis**,
With **itching**, **discharge**, and discomfort's crisis.
A **3- or 7-day cream or insert**,
To help resolve that **burn and hurt**.

It stays **local**, does not absorb,
So systemic effects are not the norm.
It's **safe in pregnancy**, usually fine —
Especially in the **second or third trimester time**.
Side effects are mild and few:
Vaginal burning, itch, odor, too.
Some may feel a bit of **cramp**,
Or **headache** if they're extra damp.

There's **no Black Box Warning** found,
But **only use vaginally**, not around.
Don't use with **tampons, douches**, or **sex**,
While on the med — just let it flex.
Contraindications? Very rare.
Just avoid with allergy care.
And not for **pediatric** use,
Unless your guidelines let it loose.

Teach to use it **right before bed**,
To keep the med where it's best spread.
And **finish the course**, even if fine,
To keep the yeast from coming in line.

TESTOSTERONE (ANDROGEL, DEPO-TESTOSTERONE)

Androgen / Hormone Replacement

When **energy dips** and **libido's low**,
Testosterone can help things flow.
It's not just "male" — in **women**, too,
It's part of what the body knew.
Used in **HRT** when levels drop,
Or **postmenopause** when drive may stop.
Also used for **gender care**,
To help align what's felt in there.

It boosts **muscle**, **bone**, and **mood**,
And helps restore **sexual attitude**.
In fertility, it plays a role,
To check if balance meets the goal.
Side effects may come to light:
Acne, hair growth, periods slight.
Voice deepening, clitoral growth,
May appear in higher dose.

Black Box Warning applies to gels:
Secondary exposure risk it tells.
Children or partners touched by skin
Can get effects they shouldn't begin.
Contraindications to know:
Pregnancy is a **firm no-go**.
Also avoid in **breast cancer space**,
Or **prostate disease** in the male race.

Teach to use it **as prescribed**,
And not to share or guess what's right.
Transdermal, IM, or buccal form,
Each one keeps their levels warm.
Use gloves if **applying gel**,
And **cover skin** — don't leave a trail.
Rotate **sites**, watch for rash,
And monitor labs to keep it on track.

TOPIRAMATE (TOPAMAX)
Anticonvulsant / Neurologic Agent

When **seizures flash** or **migraines pound**,
Topiramate helps calm things down.
It **slows the brain's electric fire**,
And calms the nerve cells wired with wire.
Used for **epilepsy** and **migraine days**,
And sometimes in **PCOS-based weight loss phase**.
Also helps with **mood swings wide**,
In **bipolar** care or **borderline** tide.

It blocks **sodium**, **glutamate**, too,
And boosts **GABA** to pull them through.
The brain gets quiet, the storm calms fast —
But side effects? Yes, they can last.
Side effects to warn up front:
Tingling hands, a **mental blunt**.
Word-finding trouble, **weight loss**, **blur**,
And **kidney stones** in those unsure.

Black Box Warning? Not on track,
But still, there's risk you must unpack:
⚠   In **pregnancy**, defects can show —
Cleft lip/palate risk may grow.
So avoid in **childbearing years**
Unless the benefits outweigh fears.

Contraindications? Not many red,
But **metabolic acidosis** must be read.
Caution with **dehydration**, too,
And avoid abrupt stops out of the blue.
Teach to drink **water** all day long,
To **prevent stones** and keep things strong.
And titrate **slow** to ease the ride,
As side effects may coincide.

It can reduce the **pill's control**,
So teach that **back-up birth** plays a role.
And don't stop suddenly — taper right,
To avoid a seizure's sudden fright.

TRANEXAMIC ACID
(LYSTEDA, CYKLOKAPRON)
Antifibrinolytic / Hemostatic Agent

When **bleeding's heavy** and won't slow down,
Tranexamic acid comes around.
It helps the **clotting stay in place**,
So flow can slow at a safer pace.
Used in **HMB** (those period floods),
Or **postpartum** when the uterus floods.
Also used in **OR bleeds**,
Where clotting support is what it needs.

It **blocks plasminogen's conversion line**,
So **fibrin clots** can hold and bind.
That stops them from **breaking down too soon**,
And helps restore the bleeding tune.
Side effects are mostly tame:
Headache, **back pain**, **cramps** to name.
Rare risks include a **clotting scare**,
So assess their history with care.

No Black Box Warning yet,
But still a **DVT risk** you must not forget.
Avoid in patients with **clotting past**,
Like **PE**, **stroke**, or **DVT cast**.
Contraindications? You bet —
Active clots, or if they sweat
A **history of hematuria** gross,
(It can worsen clots where kidneys dose).

Teach to take it **at the bleed's start**,
For periods heavy or tearing apart.
Usually taken for **up to 5 days**,
To bring that cycle back to phase.
Don't use with **hormonal birth control**
If clotting risk is on the scroll.
Monitor for **leg pain**, **vision change**,
Or anything that feels off or strange.

ULIPRISTAL ACETATE (ELLA)
Selective Progesterone Receptor Modulator (SPRM)

Ulipristal Acetate, known as **Ella**, A backup plan for any fella. When **contraception** didn't hold, She steps in brave, composed, and bold. A **SPRM**, she works so sly— She blocks **progesterone** to deny The signal that would let **eggs go**, Delaying **ovulation's** normal flow. Take it within **five days** max, After **unprotected acts**. But sooner's better—**one-pill dose**, With timing being uppermost.

It **prevents release**, not fertilized, It won't **dislodge a life inside**. So **not abortion**, as some claim— It simply keeps the egg from game.

Don't use with **ongoing hormone pills**, It may reduce how well it thrills. And don't repeat within one cycle, Or its **effectiveness may stifle**.

Side effects are mostly few— **Nausea**, **tiredness**, maybe **flu**. **Headache**, **belly pain**, or **bleeding** Can happen with the body's reading.

Tell patients that their **cycle may shift**, Their period could **delay or drift**. But if it's **more than a week late**, Test for **pregnancy**, just to be straight.

It's **contra'd in confirmed pregnancy**, And **liver disease** needs careful scrutiny. It's not for **regular birth control**, Just for when protection's stole.

CYP3A4 inducers—wait! They make it work at lower rate. So **carbamazepine**, **St. John's wort**, Might sell its **power far too short**. Though **no black box** is written down, It still requires a nursing crown. With **counseling**, and **timing taught**, We guard the risks that might be caught.

So **Ella**, with her quiet power, Protects within that fragile hour. A second chance, just one small pill— But nursing skill is vital still.

VALACYCLOVIR (VALTREX)
Antiviral / Nucleoside Analog

When **herpes flares** or **tingles brew**,
Valacyclovir pulls you through.
It's a **prodrug** turned to **acyclovir**,
That stops the virus from shifting gear.
It blocks **viral DNA synth**,
So HSV can't go to tenth.
Used for **genital herpes care**,
And to **prevent outbreaks** near labor's stare.

In **pregnancy**, it's used with pride,
At **36 weeks**, to calm the tide.
To help reduce **transmission risks**,
And **C-section plans** if lesions exist.
Also used for **shingles pain**,
Cold sores, **varicella's reign**.
But in OB, it's mainly called
When **HSV history** is installed.

Side effects are pretty chill:
Headache, **nausea**, and GI spill.
Some may feel a **dizzy zone**,
Or **fatigue** that won't leave them alone.
There's **no Black Box Warning** known,
But **renal adjustment** must be shown.
So check **creatinine** if they're frail,
To avoid a toxic trail.

Contraindications are slim:
Just **allergy to acyclovir's twin**.
And caution with **dehydration states**,
To keep the kidneys off the skates.
Teach to start it **when symptoms spark**,
Not when sores are deep and dark.
Or take it **daily** if suppressive plan,
To keep things quiet as best they can.

VENLAFAXINE (EFFEXOR, EFFEXOR XR)

SNRI (Serotonin-Norepinephrine Reuptake Inhibitor)

When **moods run low** or **hot flashes burn**,
Effexor helps the cycle turn.
Venlafaxine, a dual-track guide,
Lifts the mind while cooling the tide.
It boosts **serotonin**, and **norepinephrine**, too,
To help with **anxiety**, and **depression** in view.
But also used in **OB/GYN care**,
For **menopause** when heat fills the air.

Helps with **hot flashes, nighttime sweats**,
And mood swings some won't soon forget.
Used in women who can't take HRT,
Or want a **non-hormonal** remedy.
Taken by mouth, once or twice,
With **XR versions** that feel more nice.
Start it low, then slowly rise,
To help avoid unpleasant surprise.

Side effects? They may include:
Nausea
Dizzy,
Or **altered mood**.
⚠ **Increased BP** can sometimes show,
So **check vitals** as dosages grow.

Black box warning must be taught—
For **suicidal thoughts** that may be caught.
Especially in younger patients still,
We monitor closely and stay skillful.
Withdrawal's real, so don't stop fast,
Taper slowly so relief will last.
Teach about **timing, missed dose care**,
And when to call if symptoms flare.

Venlafaxine supports the soul,
And helps make weary women whole.
In **mental health** or **hormone tide**,
With **nursing guidance**, it walks beside.

VITAMIN D (CHOLECALCIFEROL / ERGOCALCIFEROL)

Fat-Soluble Vitamin / Hormone-Like Supplement

When **hormones shift** or **cycles stray**,
Vitamin D can light the way.
It's not just sunshine in a pill—
It fuels the womb and bones with skill.
Supports the **endometrium's glow**,
And helps the **ovaries ebb and flow**.
Linked to **fertility**, both **egg** and **sperm**,
It's a must in every OB/GYN term.

In **pregnancy**, it strengthens bones,
For **fetal growth** and **calcium zones**.
Low D may risk **preeclampsia's climb**,
Or baby's bones not forming in time.
It helps with **immunity**, keeps moods on track,
And lowers **inflammation** pushing back.
Supports those with **PCOS**,
Helping **insulin** act with less distress.

In **breastfeeding**, it fuels mom and babe,
So both stay strong from the milk she gave.
And in **perimenopause**, it plays a part—
Protecting bones and mind and heart.

Given **by mouth**, in drops or tabs,
Or **monthly high-dose** as your doc grabs.
600–2,000 IU is norm,
But check the labs to match the form.

Side effects? Rare when it's right—
But too much D can dim the light:
Hypercalcemia, thirst, or **stones**,
So don't just megadose on your own.
No black box warning, but teach the path:
To pair it with **calcium, movement**, and math.
Check **D levels** when mood feels off,
Or when bone scans make doctors scoff.

Vitamin D—more than it seems,
It's sunlight's gift behind the scenes.
With **nurse support** and tailored care,
It nurtures women everywhere.

THANK YOU

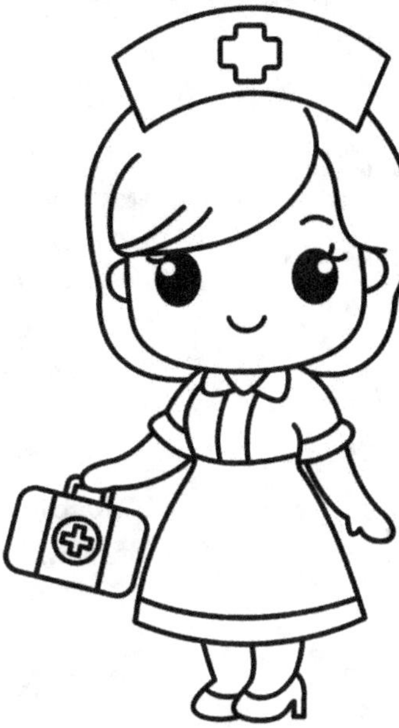

for getting this book and for making it all the way to the end!

Before you go, I wanted to ask you for one small favor. Could you please consider posting a review? Because posting a review is the best and easiest way to support the work of independent authors like me.

Your feedback will help me a ton!

Click **Here** or Scan the QR code below!

OTHER TITLES IN THE MADE EASY SERIES

Geriatrics Made Easy
Emergency Care Made Easy
Critical Care Made Easy
Human Growth & Development
Maternal & Newborn Made Easy
Mental Health Made Easy
Organic Chemistry Made Easy
General Chemistry Made Easy
Pediatrics Made Easy
Med-Surg Made Easy, Vol 1
Med-Surg Made Easy, Vol 2
Microbiology Made Easy
Nursing Skills & Procedures
Pathophysiology Made Easy
Nursing Assessment Made Easy
Nutrition Made Easy
Anatomy & Physiology Vol 1
Anatomy & Physiology Vol 2

Pharmacology Series

Pharmacology Made Easy Vol 1
Pharmacology Made Easy Vol 2
Pharmacology Made Easy Vol 3
Oncology Meds Made Easy
Cardiac Meds Made Easy
Endocrine Meds Made Easy
Pain Meds Made Easy
GI Meds Made Easy
Respiratory Meds Made Easy
Critical Meds Made Easy
ER/ICU Meds Made Easy
Neuro Meds Made Easy
Psych Meds Made Easy
Pediatric Meds Made Easy
OB/GYN Meds Made Easy

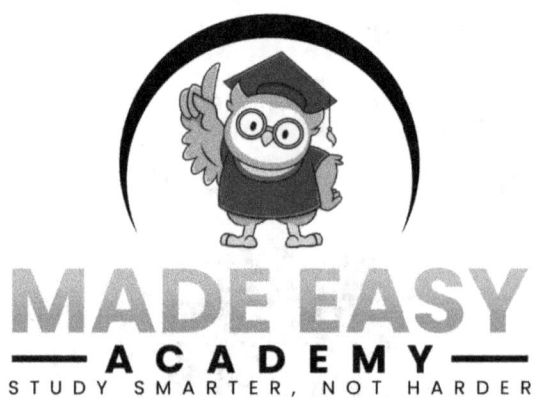

www.ingramcontent.com/pod-product-compliance
Lightning Source LLC
Chambersburg PA
CBHW071031240526
45469CB00006BD/2171